Y0-AHH-586

HEART ATTACK!

HEART ATTACK!
A Question and Answer Book

by OSCAR ROTH, M.D., F.A.C.C.

Clinical Professor of Medicine, Yale
University School of Medicine
Director, Coronary Care Unit and
Department of Electrocardiography,
Hospital of St. Raphael
Consulting Cardiologist, New Britain
General Hospital, Milford General
Hospital, West Haven Veterans Hospital,
Rocky Hill Veterans Home and Hospital

with LAWRENCE GALTON

and the editorial assistance of
William D. Roth, Ph.D.,
and Ned Thomas

J. B. LIPPINCOTT COMPANY
Philadelphia and New York

**To Stefanie, André, Bill, Evelyn, Judie, and Simone
and to the Sisters of Charity
at the HOSPITAL OF ST. RAPHAEL**

Copyright © 1978 by Oscar Roth, M.D.
All rights reserved
First edition
2 4 6 8 9 7 5 3 1
Printed in the United States of America

The illustrations in Chapter 9 are reprinted from the Supplement to the Journal of the American Medical Association, February 18, 1974. Copyright © 1974, the American Medical Association. Reprinted with permission from the American Heart Association.

The Low-Fat, Low-Cholesterol Meal Plan, Appendix E, is © reprinted with the permission of the American Heart Association.

The Mild Sodium-restricted Diet, Appendix F, is © 1969, American Heart Association, reprinted with the permission of the American Heart Association.

"If You Want to Give Up Cigarettes," Appendix G, is from the pamphlet of that name by the American Cancer Society, Inc., and is used with the Society's permission.

U.S. Library of Congress Cataloging in Publication Data

Roth, Oscar, birth date
    Heart attack!

    Includes index.
    1. Heart—Infarction—Miscellanea. I. Galton, Lawrence, joint author. II. Title. [DNLM: 1. Coronary disease—Examination questions. 2. Coronary disease—Popular works. WG18 R845h]
RC685.I6R67   616.1'23   78-500
ISBN-0-397-01263-2

Contents

Preface   13

1 Getting It Straight:
Chest Pain Versus Heart Disease   15
2 The Real Heart Pain: Angina   22
3 The Heart Attack   33
4 Afterward   59
5 Decreasing the Risks of
Occurrence and Recurrence   81
6 Tests for the Heart: What They Are,
What They Help Reveal   139
7 Heart Medications and Heart Pacemakers   150
8 Heart Surgery   177
9 Other Questions That Concern You and Your Family   187
10 Frontiers   199
11 A Parting Word   209

Glossary   211
Appendixes
   A. Desirable Weights for Men and Women   226
   B. Table of Spending Calories   227
   C. Cholesterol Content of Common Foods   228
   D. Caloric Content of Foods and Beverages   229
   E. The American Heart Association's
      Low-Fat, Low-Cholesterol Meal Plan   235
   F. Mild Sodium-restricted Diet: 1,800 Calories   241
   G. If You Want to Give Up Cigarettes   244
Index   257

Preface

The heart may be damaged in many ways: by congenital malformation, infection, inflammation, accidental injury, toxic substances such as alcohol, or atherosclerotic changes of the heart arteries (coronary artery disease).

This book will concentrate on the most common, important, and feared of all heart problems—coronary heart disease. It is also called coronary atherosclerosis or ischemic heart disease. All of us know too well that this disease is the reason for the distressing, sometimes invaliding, pain of angina and for heart attacks.

Heart attacks often occur suddenly and unexpectedly. Not uncommonly, they occur at an early age such as the mid-forties, even though the highest incidence is in the mid-sixties. They affect, and often disrupt, not only the life of the victim, but also the lives of the victim's family.

Angina pectoris—the chest pain that comes on effort, indicative of coronary heart disease—may also be devastating when severe. And even when the pain is not overwhelming, the anxiety and worry it engenders may be disruptive to the lives of the victim and his or her family.

Much confusion, much needless anxiety, and even much harm may occur because the patient and his or her family fail to obtain sufficient guidance from their physician or fail to remember everything told them after visits to the physician or after discharge from the hospital. Lack of adequate guidance can often have serious consequences for the marriage, work, quality of life, and even possibly the length of life of the angina or heart attack victim.

The purpose of this book is not to replace the personal physician's advice. On the contrary, it is to complement that advice. It should help patient and family comprehend the condition and stimulate them to ask more questions of their physician.

The questions you will find in this book are those that have been asked by patients in a long cardiology practice, and the answers are based not only on my personal experience in treating patients but also on reports in the medical literature.

I have tried to make my answers frank, revealing, and fully informative. Where there may be more than one view of an answer to the question, I have indicated that. In some areas, expert medical opinion differs, and it is helpful for you to know that; no one answer is possible at all times because medicine is still a developing art.

In the last decade, something hopeful and gratifying, even remarkable, has been happening. Although for a long time coronary heart disease has been epidemic among us, its toll in lives steadily increasing, the toll has begun to decline. Moreover, the rate of decline has been accelerating. The life expectancy of Americans has, therefore, improved. According to a U.S. Census Bureau report, it is now 81 years for women and 71.8 years for men. Less than two years ago it was 77 for women and 69.1 for men.

We now have good reason to hope that the decline in deaths from coronary heart disease will continue to accelerate—not only because of better methods of treatment (and they are indeed available now) but also because of greater understanding of the factors of the disease that cause death and of how they may be minimized or eliminated. In addition, the public, when informed, has demonstrated the capacity to respond intelligently to the possibility of reducing the risk factors.

I am grateful to the many patients who asked questions, questions that shed light on the areas puzzling and worrisome to them. I am grateful, too, to the many who helped by indicating when answers were enlightening, when they were not sufficiently so, and what was needed to make the answers useful to them.

And I owe a deep debt of gratitude to the scientists, too numerous to mention, whose work has made possible many of my answers.

1

Getting It Straight: Chest Pain Versus Heart Disease

Coronary heart disease is real enough, of course. But it can be an "un-real" problem, too. There are indications that millions of people think they have heart disease when, in fact, they do not. They may suffer some of the symptoms—most notably, chest pain—that could mean coronary heart disease but in their case do not, leading them to live needlessly anxious and limited lives.

To What Extent Are Chest Pain and Heart Disease Related?

Pain in the chest can, and often does, accompany coronary heart disease. It is, in effect, the cry of an overburdened heart having to strain too hard in the face of the disease. There are some very definite, identifying characteristics to that kind of pain, as we shall see shortly.

But not by any means does all chest pain mean something is wrong with the heart. Many conditions—a wide variety—can produce chest pain.

What Else Besides Heart Trouble Can Cause Chest Pain?

Gallbladder disease due to inflammation or stones can sometimes be mistaken for heart disease if it produces pain in the chest.

Pleurisy, an inflammation of the lining of the lungs, can also be responsible.

So can shingles, in which nerves irritated by a virus infection produce acute pain.

There is a condition called hiatus hernia—also known as diaphragmatic hernia—in which part of the stomach may protrude up through an enlarged opening in the diaphragm into the chest. A hiatus hernia may cause pain under the breastbone and the burning sensation of heartburn. The symptoms are usually worse after eating and with lifting or stooping. Sometimes the pain may resemble the chest pain associated with heart disease. An X ray can confirm the presence of hiatus hernia, and often simple measures such as elevation of the head of the bed, weight reduction, or the use of antacids can relieve the discomfort.

What Are Other Causes of Chest Pain?

Cardiospasm is an irritability of part of the esophagus, or food pipe, leading from the throat to the stomach. This condition—treatable with medication when recognized—can produce chest pain similar to that of heart disease. The pain may even radiate to the shoulders and upper arms. But cardiospastic pain has features that can distinguish it from heart pain: it is usually briefer and frequently appears during rest. However, it may initially be confused with angina, even by experienced physicians, because in some cases it can be relieved by nitroglycerin, an anti-anginal medication placed under the tongue. Careful X-ray studies help to make the right diagnosis.

Chest pain can also stem from a mild rib inflammation or from arthritis in the joints between ribs and spine or between ribs and breastbone. Tenderness on pressure differentiates such pain from angina.

It is possible, too, for shoulder bursitis, particularly when the left shoulder is affected, to produce pain similar to that of heart disease.

A condition known as the cervical root syndrome that sometimes is responsible for chest pain results from irritation or pressure affecting nerves of the neck area of the spine. The irritation may come from poor posture, from acute neck strain from a fall, or from whiplash injury. It may be caused by arthritic changes in the neck bones. One symptom of this condition may be chest pain; others may include numbness, tingling, and weakness. Posture correction sometimes is enough to help. In other cases, cervical traction, applied with a head-pulling halter or collar, may help. Medication is also sometimes beneficial. Occasionally surgery is necessary.

Chest pain can also result from an unsuspected broken rib, which might have happened during a bout of coughing.

It has even been found to be caused by food poisoning and by sleeping with arms or shoulders in an unnatural position.

And, not uncommonly, excessive air swallowing may account for worrisome chest pain.

Why Does Swallowing Air Cause Chest Pain?

Some people are accomplished, even if unknowing, air swallowers. They are "aerophagics"—literally, "air eaters."

All of us swallow air to some extent. We may swallow large amounts if we eat too fast, drink a lot of carbonated beverages, or drink liquids with a straw. But aerophagics swallow air also because they are emotionally upset. Some gastroenterologists look upon aerophagia as a nervous habit by which, as one puts it, the individual "just scratches himself with air."

Extreme aerophagia can produce symptoms alarmingly like those of serious organic troubles, as the excess air distends the stomach. In some patients, it causes discomfort much like that of gallbladder disease.

Furthermore, it can produce pain in the lower left chest that at times may be felt in the left side of the neck or left shoulder or arm—confusingly like the chest pain of heart disease. It has also been known to cause breathing difficulty, palpitation, and even a fear of impending death.

Another air-related problem—this time not excessive swallowing but rather excessive breathing—must also be considered in diagnosing chest pain.

How Does Overbreathing Produce Chest Pain?

Unusually prolonged and unusually deep breathing can accompany anxiety or emotional tension. With overbreathing—also called hyperventilation—excessive amounts of carbon dioxide are exhaled or "blown off" as large amounts of air are inhaled.

Hyperventilation leads to transient biochemical changes as a result of low body levels of carbon dioxide that can produce many symptomatic disturbances, including faintness, a feeling of tightness in the chest, a sensation of smothering, and some degree of apprehension. There may also be palpitation or pounding of the heart, a feeling of fullness in the throat, pain over the stomach region and numbness of the extremities.

In some people, hyperventilation may be responsible, with or without the presence of other symptoms, for chest pain similar to that of heart disease.

I realize it may be difficult to believe that so many disturbances can result simply from overbreathing. Yet when chest pain or any other symptom is actually due to hyperventilation, it is often possible to demonstrate the relationship clearly by having the patient deliberately overbreathe until the symptom or symptoms appear. Relief occurs when the patient then places a paper bag over nose and mouth and rebreathes in it, thus returning the level of carbon dioxide to normal. Indeed, some hyperventilators have learned to make a practice of using a paper bag for rebreathing whenever they experience an attack.

There are indications from recent research that basic to hyperventilation may be a poor-breathing habit that permits any emotional disturbance to trigger a chain reaction of excessive breathing which, in turn, may lead to more anxiety or tension and still more overbreathing.

Many people with the problem may be helped by learning to use regularly a slow diaphragmatic type of breathing, emphasizing the use of abdominal muscles and diaphragm.

It is now recognized that hyperventilation may even alter the electrocardiogram (either at rest or with exercise) and that this has led to the wrong suspicion of underlying coronary disease in many patients in the past.

Are There Emotional Causes for Chest Pain?

Without necessarily involving aerophagia or hyperventilation, emotional disturbances can be responsible for symptoms that seem like those of heart disease.

Mental depression can be a peculiar affliction. All of us have our ups and downs, days when we feel on top of the world, others when we feel a bit low. But depression—a chronic change of mood, an extended lowering of the spirits—is another matter.

It may be what is called a reactive or "exogenous" depression, meaning that it comes from outside—for example, a response to the loss of a loved one, a job, a promotion, or money.

Another common kind of depression is called "endogenous," indicating that it comes from within, with no apparent external cause. Suddenly, a person may decide that he or she is a failure in life, when that is not really true. Unaccountably, self-esteem and self-confidence vanish.

When depression occurs, it is not limited to the mind. There is a lowering of general vitality as well. And depression can produce many symptoms of seeming physical illness: headache, fatigue, sleeping disturbance (most commonly, early waking), dizziness, breathing difficulty, palpitation, nausea, chest constriction, pain in the heart area.

In fact, the physical guises of depression can be so pronounced that they overshadow the blue feelings, and when depressed people seek medical help, it is commonly for the physical disturbances, which are their main concern. The depressed feelings are often not mentioned; they seem of little consequence to the victim compared with the body symptoms. Some victims may, in fact, come to believe that their blue mood is the result, rather than the cause, of the physical disturbances.

I cannot emphasize enough how important it is that you mention the "blueness" to your physician if you have depressed feelings accompanying chest pain or any other symptoms.

Depression can be overcome, often with a brief course of drug therapy or psychotherapy or a combination of the two. And once the depression departs, so, generally, do the disturbing body symptoms.

Depression aside, an otherwise emotionally troubled person who experiences a symptom such as chest pain, breathlessness, or palpitation from any cause, including nervous upset, can all too easily develop a cardiac neurosis, becoming convinced that he or she has heart disease.

Commonly, cardiac neurotics—and they may be young adults as well as older people—become acutely aware of their heart action. With their attention unduly focused on it, they may sense disturbances in the heart's normal sounds and action. To them, it may seem to be pounding with extraordinary force, unduly loud, too rapid, or irregular, when it is actually none of these, or when their unwarranted concern and anxiety have induced such minor disturbances.

Cardiac neurotics usually are most sensitive to their heart action at night, in the quiet of their bedrooms, when they are trying to fall asleep. As a result, they may get less sleep, awaken fatigued, gather some strength as they get involved in daily activities, and then become anxious again later in the day when fatigue and exhaustion recur.

When chest pain stems from emotional problems, it can still be very real physical pain.

Are There Even More Causes?

Pain in the chest, along with one or more of a variety of other symptoms, may accompany a wide range of other conditions, among them, pneumonia, tuberculosis and other infections, emphysema, some malignancies, and ulcer of the esophagus and stomach.

What Can I Do to Find Out What Is Wrong?

If you, or any members of your family, have any symptom or set of symptoms you suspect might be caused by heart disease, do get medical help.

Don't assume that it *is* heart disease—or that it is not.

I think that after reading this book you may well come

Getting It Straight: Chest Pain Versus Heart Disease 21

away with a more precise idea of the nature of the symptoms in heart disease, with a better idea of how they may be distinguished from symptoms of other problems.

But should you decide, on your own, from the information you find here, that you do or do not have a heart problem? I urge you not to.

If, in fact, you do have heart disease, your physician can usually determine this through examination and tests, and you'll find out later in this book how he or she proceeds and why. Later you will learn that even with heart disease there are many causes of chest pain that do not stem from heart problems. Knowledge of these other causes may help you deal with them better and be less fearful of new or unusual discomforts.

If you do not have heart disease, your physician can establish what it is you do have and what to do about that.

And, if you have no serious problem at all, your physician can explain and reassure, and you will be free of needless worry and anxiety.

Not least of all, should you have coronary heart disease, there is much that can be done now to help your heart, to ease any pain, to counteract serious risk factors, and to help you live a normal life, perhaps even more active and vigorous and productive than the life you may have been leading in recent weeks, months, or years.

2

The Real Heart Pain: Angina

Chest pain can stem, as we have seen, from many problems that have nothing to do with the heart. One kind of chest pain, however, is linked to the heart. Its name: angina pectoris. *"Angina" means constricting pain; "pectoris" refers to the chest.*

What Is Angina Like?

A classic description of angina was first written more than two centuries ago, in 1768, by an English physician, William Heberden. It is vivid and concise:

> There is a disorder of the breast marked with strong and peculiar symptoms.... The seat of it, and sense of strangling, and anxiety with which it is attended, may make it not improperly be called angina pectoris. Those who are afflicted with it are seized while they are walking (more especially if it be uphill, and soon after eating) with a painful and most disagreeable sensation in the breast, which seems as if it would extinguish life if it were to increase or continue; but the moment they stand still, all this uneasiness vanishes.

Anginal pain may be felt as a viselike, constricting sensation of the whole chest or of only the area behind the breastbone in the middle of the chest. Only rarely is it restricted to just one side of the chest. Often the pain travels to the neck, jaw, lower gums, cheeks, either shoulder, arms or hands, the middle of the abdomen, or that part of the back between the shoulders.

There are variations. Occasionally, there is no chest pain, and the pain occurs only between the shoulder blades or in the left hand or wrist, left arm or shoulder, pit of the abdomen, jaws or teeth, or portions of the right arm. Sometimes the pain may go from chest to elbow or fingers. Sometimes it may start in the arm and then be felt in the chest.

When Does Angina Occur?

Usually angina occurs after such activities as walking up a hill or up stairs. It may also occur while walking on a very cold winter day or carrying a load, during sexual intercourse, while watching an exciting television program or movie, raking leaves, vacuuming, making beds, or shoveling snow, or during other strenuous activities.

In short, the pain may first be noticed under situations of strain, stress, anxiety, excitement, or effort, or after a heavy meal or in cold, windy weather.

Occasionally, a special kind of angina begins while at rest or during sleep, particularly during dreams. It may wake the patient from sleep.

Often angina is associated with a pale face or perspiration, or both.

How Long Does It Last?

Angina usually lasts from less than a minute to 10 to 20 minutes, rarely more than 20 minutes. It almost always subsides within a minute if one stops the activity associated with its onset, unless it occurs during rest or sleep.

Almost invariably, an angina attack compels you to stop whatever you are doing; it's frightening as well as painful. The short, extremely frightening nature of the discomfort is a hallmark of angina.

Another hallmark is what you are likely to do if asked to

point to where the pain is. Hardly ever does anyone with angina point to the involved area with a finger or two. Instead, the patient is likely to point with a clenched fist, an entire open hand, or both hands or fists.

Where Does the Trouble Lie?

As I indicated earlier (Chapter 1), the pain in the chest—the anginal pain—that accompanies coronary heart disease is, in effect, the protesting cry of an overburdened heart having to strain too hard in the face of the disease.

The trouble lies with the nourishment supply for the heart. Though sufficient under routine circumstances, the supply isn't adequate when there is a special demand on the heart because of vigorous activity or any kind of stress or strain.

In a way, it's like a car that moves along well on level stretches but then falters while climbing a hill. Its engine sputters as a result of not getting enough gas, because the gas-supply line is too narrowed to meet the increased fuel demand for climbing. When angina appears, it's because the heart's supply lines have been affected. The coronary arteries, which feed the heart itself with nourishing blood, have been attacked, narrowed—their blood-carrying capacity diminished—by a process called atherosclerosis.

The next few pages give some basic information on the heart and its circulation and on the process and effects of atherosclerosis.* It can be most helpful to you in understanding not only angina but also the treatment and prevention of heart attack—what physicians can do and what you can do.

About the size of your fist and weighing less than a pound, the heart is a tough muscular organ. It pumps huge amounts of blood through the body—the entire 7-quart content once through the body every 80 seconds. Daily, it pumps the equiva-

---

*If you are thoroughly familiar with this, you may wish to turn to the next question.

lent of about 5,500 quarts weighing 6 tons through the body's miles of blood vessels.

It has four chambers: two for receiving blood and two for pumping it. The two upper, receiving chambers are called atria or auricles; the two lower, pumping chambers are called ventricles.

Into the atrium on the right side of the heart comes blood that has circulated through the body and given up its oxygen. When the right atrium fills, it contracts to pass the blood through a valve into the right ventricle below. And the right ventricle contracts to propel the blood into the pulmonary artery, which, through its branches, carries it to both lungs. There, the blood delivers up its cargo of carbon dioxide and takes on a fresh cargo of oxygen.

From the lungs the freshened blood moves through pulmonary veins into the left atrium on the other side of the heart. As the atrium fills, it contracts to send the blood through a valve into the left ventricle below.

Contracting powerfully, the left ventricle then pumps the blood into the aorta. This is the body's great trunk-line artery, with a diameter about equal to that of a large garden hose. From the aorta many arteries branch off to take fresh blood to all parts of the body.

As you can see, then, the heart is not really one pump but two: one to push blood to the lungs to be refreshed, the other to push the oxygen-rich freshened blood out to the body. Both pumps work in concert, with the atria almost simultaneously receiving blood from body and lungs, and the ventricles almost simultaneously contracting and pumping.

The normal heart is remarkably adaptive. Under resting conditions the ventricles pump out, with each contraction, only slightly more than half the blood they contain. That's adequate for body needs. But when the body needs more—when you exercise, for example—the ventricles can contract harder to pump out their total content. And the heart rate can speed up also, to meet increased body needs so that there are more frequent as well as more forceful contractions per minute.

What sets the heart rate? A pacemaker, which is an area of special tissue inside the right atrium, gets signals from centers in the brain and spinal cord that are sensitive to the body's varying needs under different circumstances. It also reacts to hormones released by the adrenal and thyroid glands.

In response, the pacemaker sends out tiny electrical signals that cause the atria to force blood into the ventricles and, in turn, the ventricles to propel the blood out.

The heart is an unusual muscle, working away at about 70 beats a minute, day and night, for a lifetime. Like any muscle, it requires nourishment, and for that it depends on its own special coronary circulation rather than on the blood passing through the heart chambers.

The coronary circulation system consists of two coronary arteries which, like arteries that supply other parts of the body, branch off from the great aorta.

The coronaries run down the front and back of the heart and divide into branches, as do other arteries in the body. The branches divide and subdivide so that they cover the back as well as the front of the heart.

Just as the heart adapts to body needs, so does the coronary circulation.

Under resting conditions, the coronary arteries receive from the aorta an amount of blood sufficient for the heart's needs. When the heart has to work harder, beating more often and more powerfully, it needs more nourishment and the coronaries receive more blood from the aorta.

You may remember seeing in the past the word *arteriosclerosis*. It means artery hardening. Coronary artery disease, which used to be called coronary arteriosclerosis, is now known as *atherosclerosis*. *Athero* means soft swelling. Atherosclerosis is a more accurate term because coronary artery disease starts with a soft swelling of the artery's inner lining and progresses to hardening.

When atherosclerosis begins to develop, the first visible indication may be a fatty streak in the inside lining of an artery, a thin, yellowish, slightly raised line. It may be no more than half an inch long, and an eighth of an inch wide.

As atherosclerosis progresses, the streak increases in size

and becomes the typical "plaque" of the disease. A plaque is filled with fatty material. In its early stages when it is still small and soft, it may heal over and disappear. As a plaque grows in size, with time, calcium may be deposited in it, making it hard. Then it does not go away.

The process of plaque development is slow. And not all portions of the coronary arteries are affected equally. Some may remain clear; others may have many plaques.

As plaques enlarge, they begin to stick out into the lumen, or channel, of the artery, much as do scales forming within a corroding pipe.

Now you can begin to visualize what may happen.

A healthy coronary artery is relatively small. It has a diameter of about 2 to 3 millimeters, or $2/25$ to $3/25$ inch. A wooden match stick would fit snugly inside.

As atherosclerosis progresses, with the plaques enlarging and thus shrinking the internal diameter of an artery, there may be no symptoms for years. Enough blood flows through to meet the needs of the heart.

But at some point during the progression of the disease the channel within the artery may be so narrowed and the blood flow reduced just enough to bring on the first attack of angina pectoris. This usually occurs when the original diameter of the artery is reduced by more than 75 percent.

The first attack may come while climbing a flight of stairs, running to catch a bus, shoveling snow, playing tennis, [or] even just breasting a cold wind or after any kind of excitement.

Under those circumstances of strain, once taken in stride, the flow is no longer adequate to meet the heart's increased needs. The extra surge can't get through the narrowed vessel.

And the heart protests.

Pain anywhere in the body has a purpose—to alert you to a danger. Touch a hot stove and the pain provides a sharp warning that makes you withdraw your finger before it is burned severely.

The heart's protest—anginal pain—is an unmistakable alert signal that what you're doing is too much. You stop it. With the excess demand on the heart removed, the angina goes away.

Does Angina Always Accompany Atherosclerosis?

No.

There can be great differences in the way different people are affected by coronary atherosclerosis.

Even with advanced disease, some people live long and active lives without ever experiencing angina, and when they die at eighty or even later it may be from something having nothing to do with the heart: cancer, an accident, an infection.

The reason seems to be that they, fortunately, develop collateral circulation—new blood routes that connect between coronary branches, bypassing diseased and blocked sections and getting adequate blood supply to the heart muscle.

Many, however, are less fortunate. They may experience angina in their forties and fifties, or even earlier.

Sometimes a heart attack may be the very first indication of coronary disease (although, looking back, there may have been warning signs falsely interpreted as indigestion, gas, or chest pressure).

How Would I Know I Have Atherosclerosis If I Don't Have Angina?

Because symptoms may not be obvious, you should have periodic examinations by your physician.

In a physical examination, perhaps coupled with laboratory and other tests, your physician may discover a heart condition in the absence of any discomfort or other indication of which you're aware. Early treatment can then be started.

You—and your physician—can be particularly watchful if certain risk factors are present.

One of these risk factors is elevated blood pressure—hypertension. Another is excess weight. And others include elevated blood lipids or fats, excessive smoking, diabetes mellitus, sedentary living, personality factors that cause stress, and possibly excess uric acid in the blood. We'll be considering these and other risk factors in Chapter 5.

As I Grow Older, Is Atherosclerosis More Likely to Be Present?

It may be more advanced.

Atherosclerosis, we know now, usually becomes more severe with the passing of years—in some people even more so and at an earlier age than in others. But it doesn't develop, to begin with, simply because of time.

That was once thought to be the case. But the notion that atherosclerotic disease was associated only with aging was jolted during World War II. During the war, physicians began to note heart attacks in relatively young men in the armed forces. They gathered information on 866 cases of heart attack in men ages eighteen through thirty-nine. Most had been in apparent good health until the very moment of attack. Sixty-four of the men were less than twenty-four years old; more than 200 of the total of 866 were under twenty-nine. And when physicians studied the coronary arteries in the young men who died, they found the typical changes of atherosclerosis.

Still other evidence that atherosclerosis is not only associated with advancing age came during the Korean War. Physicians performed postmortem studies on many soldiers killed in battle. The average age of these men was twenty-two years. Yet when the coronary arteries were opened and examined, atherosclerosis was found to be present.

Despite seemingly good health, artery disease had begun. In 10 percent of these very young men, the atherosclerotic process had already narrowed, by 70 percent or more, the channel in one or both coronary arteries.

In one way, of course, these were disturbing studies. But in another very significant way they were constructive.

By underscoring the fact that atherosclerosis is not something inevitable with age—something therefore unassailable—the studies focused attention on what factors other than age might be involved in starting up the disease and causing it to progress. This led to an understanding of the risk factors we will be talking about later.

Is a Woman as Likely to Be Affected as a Man?

Women are by no means exempt from atherosclerosis. The magnitude of the problem in men—particularly of one of the end results, heart attack—has tended somewhat to obscure its importance in women.

Yet the fact is that coronary heart disease has been accounting for more than 200,000 deaths a year among American women, a death toll 60 percent greater than that from cancer.

Up to the age of forty-five, men have thirteen times as many attacks as do women. Between that age and age sixty-two, men still have more—about twice as many more. But after the age of sixty-two, women are just as susceptible. Recent studies indicate that some younger women, particularly some who smoke and/or use oral contraceptives, may have increased susceptibility.

What Other Arteries Beside Those of the Heart May Be Affected by Atherosclerosis? And with What Symptoms and Results?

Atherosclerosis may affect other blood vessels: those serving the kidneys, intestines, brain, and legs.

It is likely to be present and developing for many years before producing symptoms.

When the leg arteries are involved, the patient may eventually experience pain in the hip or calf while walking, with the pain disappearing at rest. This is called claudication.

When vessels nourishing the brain are involved, there may be some degree of impairment of brain function, affecting speech, vision, coordination, or balance. Just as a heart attack may occur when atherosclerosis in a coronary artery has progressed to the point of allowing blood flow to a portion of the heart to be cut off, so may a *stroke* occur when the same disease advances to a similar point in a brain artery. As you know, weakness or paralysis of one side of the body—fortunately often only temporary—may follow a stroke.

If kidney arteries are involved, *high blood pressure* or slowly progressive kidney disease and failure may result.

Moreover, atherosclerosis of the arteries that supply blood

The Real Heart Pain: Angina

to the intestinal tract may cause abdominal pain after meals. This pain is called abdominal angina.

(Let me add here that the outlook for people with atherosclerosis affecting these other vessels as well as for those with coronary disease is far from hopeless. In fact, excellent results (discussed in Chapter 8) are now being obtained in many cases with surgery in which vessels made of dacron and other materials are implanted to bypass blocked or weakened areas. In some cases, blocked vessels may be reamed out to restore an open inner channel for blood flow.)

If I Have Any Doubt as to Whether or Not I Am Experiencing Angina, Can a Physician Diagnose It?

Yes.

As we noted earlier, chest pains can stem from many things—some of them quite simple—having nothing to do with the heart. So if you suspect you might possibly have angina but can't be certain, it's no indication of stupidity. Understandably enough, many people are confused.

To reach a diagnosis of angina, your physician will take a detailed history and ask you to describe as best you can the symptoms you experience and under what circumstances. A careful physical examination will be made, including listening to your heart. Your physician may also take an electrocardiogram (ECG). An electrocardiogram taken while you are at rest may provide an indication of coronary artery disease. (We will discuss this test in some detail in Chapter 6.)

In many cases, a resting ECG in a person with angina isn't enough; it provides no clue. Then, your physician may take another ECG reading—this time after you perform some standard exercise such as moving up and down a little set of stairs or walking fast on a treadmill. An exercise ECG often helps in the diagnosis of angina.

It's very likely that as the result of history, examination, and testing your physician can tell you whether or not you have angina.

If there should still be any question, a useful means of confirming the presence of angina is to have you try the effect of a nitroglycerin pill. (We will be considering nitroglycerin—what it is and what it does—in Chapter 7.) In angina, nitroglycerin usually relieves pain within one to three minutes. It may do so in a few other conditions causing chest pain, and in itself is not diagnostic of angina, but it is helpful in combination with the other procedures I've mentioned.

Isn't the Pain of Angina Much Like That of a Heart Attack? Does It Differ in Any Way? How Can I Know Which Is Which?

The pain of a heart attack may be very similar to that of angina.

Angina is usually triggered by physical exertion, cold air, or emotional disturbance, although it sometimes occurs at rest. A heart attack can also be precipitated by unusual physical or emotional stress, although it too may occur during rest and even during sleep.

An angina patient who suffers a heart attack may assume at first that this is angina again. But this time stopping activity doesn't work as it does for angina; the chest pain continues. This time, too, nitroglycerin doesn't relieve the pain as it does with anginal pain.

Typically, the pain that occurs with a heart attack—it may range from a feeling of pressure to a feeling that the chest is being crushed in a vise—lasts for hours and does not subside until a narcotic such as morphine is administered.

So if you have angina and have been under medical treatment for it, and are using nitroglycerin pills, you can suspect—and should suspect in order to be safe—that you are experiencing a heart attack if stopping anything you have been doing doesn't help and if the symptoms persist even after the third nitroglycerin pill.

And if you have not experienced angina before, you may suspect—and, here again, should suspect in order to be safe—that you are experiencing a heart attack if you get sudden chest pain and stopping whatever you have been doing doesn't help.

Heart attack symptoms and what happens in a heart attack will be discussed more fully in the next chapter.

3

The Heart Attack

During the course of any hour, day and night, 125 men and women in the United States experience heart attacks—two every minute. What are the symptoms? What happens to the body? If you suffer—or suspect you may be suffering—an attack, what should you do? What can be done for you? What will happen—what will your minutes, hours, days be like?

Are There Particular Times of Day—And Special Circumstances—Under Which Heart Attacks Occur?

No. They can occur at any hour and under varying circumstances—in the midst of a hard set of tennis, while running to catch a bus, while shoveling snow, or in the middle of a heated argument, but also while you're having a pleasant dinner or resting or sleeping.

Is It Possible to Have a Mild Heart Attack Without Realizing It?

Yes. What are called "silent" heart attacks do occur occasionally.

Sometimes, during a routine examination, a physician will find evidence of a past heart attack in an electrocardiogram. Yet, the patient has no memory of an attack. And, in fact, the episode may have been relatively minor, the heart muscle so little affected, that no symptoms at all occurred.

Some so-called silent attacks, however, are not really silent. They do produce symptoms but the symptoms may be mild or may be misinterpreted.

A patient with an electrocardiogram showing an unrecognized heart attack in the past may sometimes recall having had a bad case of indigestion, or a pain in an arm or in the neck thought to be a muscle cramp. Or there may be a memory of having felt extremely tired and taking longer than usual to regain strength.

But such attacks are not common. Usually a heart attack makes itself known by its symptoms.

How Can a Heart Attack Usually Be Recognized?

Chest pain is by far the most common symptom. At times, it may be localized in the upper-mid abdomen.

The pain can vary greatly in severity. On the one hand, it can be a slight feeling of pressure, of oppression in the chest. At the other extreme, it can be very severe, crushing, viselike, sometimes spreading into the throat, the shoulders, the arms, even the back.

Some people are prostrated immediately. Others walk around trying to find relief.

As we noted earlier, if a person has had anginal pain in the past and then experiences a heart attack, he or she may think at first that the chest pain is angina again. But the chest pain of a heart attack does not stop, does not respond to rest or to nitroglycerin. Often, it may even begin at rest. It may radiate to the neck, jaw, right or left shoulder or arm, or to the region between the shoulders in the back. Occasionally, the pain will not be in the chest, only in the area of radiation.

Are There Other Symptoms with the Pain?

Commonly there is a feeling of great anxiety, even of impending death. Also, there is often a cold sweat and the face turns almost gray.

The Heart Attack

There may be retching, belching, or vomiting and sometimes these may cause a heart attack to be confused with a stomach upset.

Shortness of breath is not inevitable, but it is common. Sometimes a patient will gasp for air during an attack. In some cases, there are palpitations—sensations that the heart is beating abnormally hard and fast.

What Steps Should Be Taken Immediately?

Get medical help. Dial your local emergency telephone number. Always have it readily available. If there is no such number, call the fire department, rescue squad, or ambulance. If you can't get an immediate response, get to the emergency room of the nearest hospital on your own or any other way you can.

Why Is Immediate Medical Attention So Important?

There is only one safe way to tell what is causing your chest pain or other symptoms: have a physician check right away.

Medical attention without delay can be absolutely vital. In some cases, a few minutes have meant the difference between life and death—which is why most physicians urge patients to go immediately to the hospital rather than wait for medical help at home.

Far more often than not, heart attacks don't have to be fatal. Many who die from an attack die needlessly. They die, even though, despite their attack, their hearts are too good to die—that is, the damage to the heart muscle is not enough to cause death.

More than 80 percent of heart attack deaths occur within the first twenty-four hours, many within the first hour. You might expect that extensive damage to the heart accounts for the deaths. But in many victims of a fatal heart attack, the heart is only minimally damaged. Sudden death after a heart attack is somewhat comparable to the way a clock sometimes stops ticking even though its mechanism is still in good working order.

Why does a heart that is still basically sound and too good

to die stop? Electrical failure. I'll be discussing that further with you shortly.

But for right now, let me make this point: Electrical failure of the heart can often be prevented from happening—and, if it should happen, can often be overcome—when the patient gets immediate medical attention.

So if you know you're experiencing a heart attack, or have only the slightest suspicion that you may be, get to an emergency room. At once.

Once you're there, waste no time in saying that you may be having a heart attack. That will get you immediate and appropriate attention.

Delay by heart attack victims in getting medical attention is awesomely common. The following information will help show how important prompt action is.

More than half of the 600,000 people who die each year of heart attacks succumb before they reach a hospital, where their chances for survival would have been greatly improved.

When University of Rochester cardiologists did a special study of coronary patients to find out how much time had elapsed between onset of symptoms and hospitalization, the average interval turned out to be 3½ hours. In some cases, the delay stretched for as long as five days. Transportation time to the hospital accounted for only a tiny fraction of the delay—20 minutes on average.

The trouble was that patients were slow to seek help even when symptoms should have been unmistakable. Eighty percent had experienced intense chest pain, yet had delayed seeking help.

In another study to determine what delaying patients had mistakenly thought was wrong, many were found to have initially attributed their symptoms to gas pains, some to colds, still others to gallbladder disease. Another study showed much the same mistaken notions, with a few victims believing they might have a lung condition.

Still other studies have looked into the circumstances that

The Heart Attack

determine which heart attack victims delay seeking help and under what circumstances.

Older people hesitate more often than younger. In one study, patients over seventy waited an average of 5.8 hours before deciding to get help; those under fifty sought help much sooner on the average.

People delay longer when they're alone than when they're with someone. A spouse nearby cuts the waiting time greatly.

Decision time shortens if an attack occurs at night. It lengthens if the patient takes an over-the-counter medicine such as an antacid for his pain. Only 10 percent of patients who reached a hospital in less than an hour had such medication, one study found, while 41 percent of those who got help only after a delay of twelve hours or more had used a patent medicine. People also tend to delay longer on weekends than they do during the week.

At a special American College of Cardiology conference on the delay problem, experts agreed that heart attack victims often hold off seeking help—and even deny to themselves and others that they have symptoms of an attack—because they believe that a heart attack is a completely incapacitating condition from which they will never truly recover.

But that is wrong. A heart attack victim reaching a hospital quickly after an attack begins not only has an excellent prospect of leaving the hospital alive but also a very good and constantly improving likelihood that he or she will be able to return to a full life, including work, sex, and play.

What Happens in the Body to Cause a Heart Attack?

Although a heart attack occurs suddenly, it is really the long-term result of a slowly developing disease process—the process called atherosclerosis we talked about earlier.

Over an extended period of years, as fatty deposits are laid down on the inner wall of a coronary artery, the channel for blood flow slowly narrows.

At the same time, some scarlike tissue forms and projects

into the channel and the bloodstream. Such projections may encourage some clotting of the blood. There may be tiny clots that cause no problems, but if a large clot should form in a narrow artery it may block the blood flow.

Sometimes a fatty deposit on the artery wall will rupture. This may happen during severe exertion, which leads to a rise of pressure within a diseased coronary artery. The ruptured material may then move in the bloodstream, arriving at a site in a smaller coronary vessel or branch where it may produce a blockage.

Emotional stress can lead to increased secretion of body chemicals called catecholamines. These may favor development of a clot.

For whatever reason, when a coronary vessel becomes blocked, a heart attack follows. A part of the heart muscle ordinarily supplied by blood flowing through that vessel no longer gets nourishment. Lacking the vital supply of blood and its content of oxygen, that part of the heart begins to ache—and that is the pain experienced in a heart attack.

Are Some Attacks More Serious Than Others? How So?

The severity of an attack depends on the particular artery that has become plugged.

If it is a major artery, upon which a large portion of the heart muscle depends for its blood supply, then the attack is severe. If the plugged artery is a small one, the attack may be relatively minor.

Does the Severity of Symptoms Indicate the Severity of the Attack?

Not necessarily. It's possible to have relatively less severe symptoms with a very severe attack, and relatively more severe ones with a milder attack.

The Heart Attack

How Can the Severity Be Determined?

An immediate determination of the severity is not always possible.

Many factors enter into the severity of the heart attack and these can be tested for and the severity then established.

A series of electrocardiograms taken at intervals provides a clue. Also, when heart tissue is damaged an excess of certain enzymes is released by that tissue into the blood, and these enzymes can be measured to add another clue.

The degree and duration of fever, the white blood cell count, and the blood pressure also enter into the picture. In addition, a patient's progress counts very much in assessing severity.

As you see, it is possible to measure the severity of heart attacks along many dimensions. One person's heart attack may be worse than someone else's in one way, but better in another respect.

Obviously it's useless to try to compare the severity of one's own heart attack to that of a friend or neighbor. The recuperative power of the heart and the medical care one receives can greatly influence the course of the recovery after an attack, and these factors may, in fact, considerably reduce the severity.

If There Is Damage to the Heart, Why Isn't a Heart Attack Always Fatal?

Because the heart has capacity to spare.

It isn't unique in that. You can, for example, live with only one of your two kidneys, if necessary—and many people do. Similarly, you can live, and often live well, if you have to lose part of a lung or even a whole lung.

The heart is intrinsically tough—remarkably so. It has to be in order to beat some 100,000 times a day, nearly 40 million times a year. It's more efficient than any machine yet devised by man. The work it does is comparable to the effort you would have to make to lift a ten-pound weight three feet off the ground twice a minute for the whole of your life. It produces so much energy that if its lifetime output were concentrated into one burst of power it could lift a battleship several feet out of the water.

Unless a huge amount of heart muscle is destroyed in an attack—and that is the exception, not the rule—the remaining healthy heart muscle can usually function effectively.

What's the Immediate Prime Danger?

The electrical failure I mentioned just briefly before.

Usually, early death from a heart attack is not caused by or related to the amount of heart muscle destroyed. Instead, death is usually caused by disturbance in the heart rhythm.

Even slight damage to the heart muscle may set up electrical conduction disturbances.

You'll recall that earlier (in Chapter 2) we noted that a pacemaker area in one part of the heart sends out electrical signals that govern the heart's rhythmic beating. The signals, of course, travel through the heart muscle tissue. They follow conduction paths.

With damage to the heart muscle, there may be an upset in the electrical conduction. The heart rhythm then can become abnormal. There can be very rapid beating of the ventricles, the heart's pumping chambers. Called ventricular tachycardia, that kind of beating may, in a short period of time, turn into ventricular fibrillation—a useless twitching or quivering instead of beating—which can progress to cardiac arrest, complete failure of the heart to pump blood.

That's the big problem—electrical disturbance. It usually happens early in a heart attack, if it happens at all.

But these disturbances can be treated successfully if treatment can be given in time. They can be treated at the scene of the heart attack by specially trained ambulance attendants. They can be treated by doctors and nurses in a hospital's emergency room, in the coronary care unit, and in the wards of a hospital.

I'll give you some more facts later in this chapter about how the treatment is carried out—how it's possible not only to stop fibrillation and restore normal rhythm when electrical fail-

The Heart Attack

ure has gone that far, but also to prevent it from going that far in the first place.

What Will Happen Should I Enter the Hospital with a Heart Attack?

Without delay, indicate you think you may be having a heart attack. That, as I noted earlier, will get you prompt attention, which is essential.

The physician in charge, notified that there is the possibility of an attack, will see you, ask you questions about your complaints, the symptoms you're experiencing. He or she will be trying to determine whether you are really having a heart attack or have some other condition.

But the physician will not wait to arrive at a complete diagnosis before getting you ready for treatment for a heart attack. As soon as there is cause for *suspicion* of an attack, you will receive medication to ease your discomfort. You will be administered oxygen either by mask or through a nasal tube.

A plastic tube and needle from a bottle containing glucose (sugar) solution will be connected to a vein. With that connection in place, if it should become necessary to administer medication quickly it can simply be injected into the tube. Administration of medicine directly into the bloodstream brings quickest action. It takes a drug only seconds to go from a vein in your arm to your heart.

Will All This Happen in the Emergency Room?

And more.

An electrocardiogram will be taken. Usually, this will reveal or suggest the presence of a heart attack. But occasionally, in less than 2 percent of patients, the first electrocardiogram will be normal despite the presence of an attack.

A chest X ray may be taken to determine the size of your heart. The X ray is useful, too, for determining whether your heart is still strong enough, can pump adequately enough, to remove all the fluid from your lungs. At times, the X ray may reveal other causes of chest pain, such as a collapsed lung (pneumothorax) or a blood clot in a lung (pulmonary embolus).

During a heart attack, enzymes from damaged heart tissue enter your bloodstream. Blood tests will be carried out to see if such enzymes are present. If they are typically elevated in the blood, it is probable confirmation that you are indeed having a heart attack.

And, hardly least of all, so that your heart rhythm can be checked continuously, electrodes will be placed on your body and connected with a monitor that displays the functioning of your heart. This monitor is invaluable. It helps to detect *instantly* any irregularity that may occur in your heart rhythm. If an irregularity does occur, appropriate medication can be administered easily, almost instantly, through the tubing already connected to your vein. Don't try to diagnose such irregularities yourself. They're too complicated unless you're trained to understand and deal with them. Watching the monitor may only frighten you needlessly; avoid watching.

How Long Will I Be in the Emergency Room?

Perhaps half an hour or so—a busy half hour. Cooperate completely in all these procedures.

Expect a certain degree of dispatch—indeed, sometimes brusqueness—which is necessary in the case of a heart attack.

What Will Happen Next?

If after the first half hour or so it's clear—or even if there is any suspicion—that you are having a heart attack, you will probably be transferred to a coronary care unit.

What Will Happen in the Coronary Care Unit?

An area set aside for the exclusive care of heart attack patients, the coronary care unit is specially equipped and staffed

THE HEART ATTACK

with nurses specially trained in caring for cardiac patients. Cardiologists, or heart specialists, are on call, and your own physician will have been notified.

In the coronary care unit—the CCU, as it is commonly called—you will be connected to monitors. Your heartbeat will be continuously relayed to a viewing screen in the nurses' station nearby.

If any abnormality should develop in your heart action, the staff will be instantly aware of the change. Choosing from a variety of medications and equipment, they can immediately treat you and usually restore normal rhythm.

Since the advent of coronary care units, the survival rate of acute heart attack patients has increased markedly; in most hospitals, it is over 85 percent; before 1965 it was *under* 75 percent. Where 30 of every 100 patients formerly died, now less than 15 of every 100 do so—a death reduction of 50 percent.

If I Develop a Rhythm Abnormality How Will I Be Treated?

If it's a severe abnormality—fibrillation—and it causes you to lose consciousness, metal plates will be placed against your chest and a carefully calibrated electric charge delivered to shock your heart back to normal rhythm.

More likely, you won't need that. An early, far less severe, rhythm abnormality—one which precedes fibrillation—probably will become apparent and will be overcome with drugs.

Here I think it will be helpful to you to have an understanding of what can be done to treat abnormal rhythms and to prevent the severe ones from occurring. And perhaps a particularly good, clear, concise way of providing that is to let you see how present treatments—and even the CCU itself—came about.*

Quick, effective treatment for heart-rhythm abnormalities after a heart attack—even the worst, potentially fatal ones—and for preventing lesser arrhythmias from progressing to the worst

---

*If you're already familiar with this, you can skip to the next question.

has become available only in recent years, after many years of research laid the groundwork for it.

As we have seen, the potentially lethal abnormal rhythm that may develop in a heart attack is ventricular fibrillation, in which the heart, no longer contracting at all, becomes a quivering mass.

As far back as the turn of the century, some pioneering physiologists in Switzerland discovered that they could induce ventricular fibrillation in dogs and then quickly overcome it and get the heart beating normally again if they applied strong electric currents to the heart through the opened chest.

It was thirty years before a Johns Hopkins University engineering professor, William B. Kouwenhoven, devised a practical device that could deliver current to a human heart in fibrillation. Some years after that, at Harvard, Dr. Paul M. Zoll found that it wasn't necessary to open the chest and apply the current directly to the heart; the shock could be delivered effectively through the chest wall. Still later, in 1960, Dr. Bernard Lown and a Harvard team made a significant advance—with a way of delivering a single electrical pulse that was far more effective than earlier devices.

Even so, few victims of fibrillation could be helped. All too rarely was it possible to get the equipment to a victim in time. With fibrillation, there is no more blood circulation. The heart is just quivering, not pumping. For lack of blood, serious brain damage can develop within three or four minutes after fibrillation begins. And for lack of blood, too, the already damaged heart muscle is further damaged—to the point where in a few minutes after fibrillation starts, the heart, no matter how much shocked, cannot resume normal beating.

In the face of this, Kouwenhoven, the engineer, working with Dr. James Jude, had another contribution to make. He was able to show that, in a person whose heart has stopped beating, compressing the lower part of the breastbone could actually move enough blood to keep the heart, brain, and other vital organs alive, allowing time to get equipment to the bedside.

But it was to be the coronary care unit and the well-equipped ambulance that would make possible the saving of many lives—in more ways than one.

In their first efforts, the CCUs saved lives through resuscitation. If you go into fibrillation and can be treated within just one minute, you have a 90 percent, or even greater, chance of living. But if there is a three-minute delay you have much less of a chance.

In a CCU, you can be treated easily within a minute. The equipment is immediately at hand. There is no need even to wait for a physician if one is not immediately available. Nurses are trained to place the paddles of the defibrillator, as the equipment is called, on your chest and administer the one or more pulses of current needed to get the heart back into normal rhythm. While waiting for the defibrillator to be wheeled to the bedside, a single fist blow from a distance of about one foot over the middle portion of the breastbone may restore regular rhythm.

But CCUs have gone well beyond resuscitation alone.

Does ventricular fibrillation develop suddenly? Yes, but not without advance warning—if that warning can be noted. And if you're in a CCU that warning can be noted and noted quickly.

Most of the time, fibrillation is preceded by lesser rhythm abnormalities—and those abnormalities can be detected. They give warning, in fact, on the monitor in the nurses' station. And when the warning comes, the nurses know exactly what to do—with or without the help of a physician.

Drug treatment for the lesser rhythm abnormality commonly can prevent fibrillation from coming on.

One of many drugs that may be used, for example, is lidocaine. This is the same compound used by dentists as a local anesthetic. It also acts as an anti-arrhythmia agent. It can be infused continuously into a vein in tiny amounts for forty-eight hours or longer until an abnormal rhythm disappears.

Hospitals that have kept long-term records have found that whereas almost one in every six heart-attack patients formerly developed fibrillation, now it occurs in less than one in fifty cases.

What Else Will Be Done?

Oxygen may be administered, when necessary. It may be used if you have some difficulty breathing, for just a short time for several days.

When you get oxygen a rich supply enters the blood and reaches the heart muscle. Oxygen also helps to ease breathing and may diminish pain and aid sleep.

What About Pain?

The initial pain will be eased for you with a pain-relieving drug. If necessary, a narcotic may be used at first to assure relief. It won't be needed for long and you don't have to worry at all about becoming addicted.

In rare circumstances when pain persists despite all medication, a special device called an intra-aortic balloon can be inserted into a leg artery and often relieves pain. Rhythmically inflated and deflated by a machine, it helps improve blood flow in the coronary arteries and decrease the work of the heart. Thus, at once, it increases oxygen supply and decreases the amount of oxygen needed. The oxygen deficit and the pain caused by it are improved.

After the initial pain begins to disappear, you may occasionally experience a new sort of pain, particularly when you breathe in. If it occurs, it usually does so from the second to the fourth day after a heart attack.

The pain is not a sign of a new heart attack or of angina. Rather, it results from a harmless, self-limiting localized inflammation of the pericardium, the sac around the heart, called *ischemic pericarditis.* "Ischemic" indicates deficiency of blood and oxygen in an area, and the ending "itis" in the word pericarditis means inflammation.

This pain will gradually subside by itself. Should it prove too uncomfortable, signal for the nurse. It will quickly respond to aspirin or other medication.

Will I Be Sedated?

You may be—for good reason.

It's only natural for you to feel some anxiety after a heart attack. It's the rare patient who does not.

As you know, anxiety—and anger, fear, and other emotions—have effects on the body. Undoubtedly, nature intended them to. They alert the body and ready it for physical action. The readiness takes many forms—tensing of muscles, quicker breathing, increased gland secretions, faster heartbeat—all designed to let you fight or flee in the face of a danger or a challenging situation.

Especially immediately after a heart attack, emotional upset should be avoided if at all possible, in order to spare the heart the extra burden. Sedation can be helpful in minimizing the stress of anxiety on the heart.

Sedation aside, you can do much to reduce the stress if you talk about your anxiety with your physician, bringing your thoughts and feelings out in the open. Anxiety after a heart attack commonly stems from a patient's lack of knowledge of what has happened, what is being done for him and why, what will happen next, whether he is progressing well or badly, what the future holds.

The more you know about all these things, the less likely by far that you will be unduly, upsettingly anxious.

I hope that what we are discussing here will be helpful in this respect. I hope, too, that you will talk with your physician and ask questions that are bothering you. It is very likely that he or she can reassure you that you are progressing, will recover, and will *not* be an invalid or anything approaching it. Experience in the past decade has shown that the majority of heart-attack victims return to normal, productive lives.

What About My Diet?

It's likely to be light for the first few days. Perhaps only broth, fruit juice, tea. The less you have to digest, the less work for the heart.

Later, you'll get the nourishment you need in the form of light meals, possibly four or five a day, rather than three larger ones.

How Long Will I Be Flat on My Back?

Not long—not nearly as long as you might suppose. And not nearly as long as once was customary.

Your heart, of course, has suffered some damage. Since it has to go on beating and pumping blood, it can't have complete rest. But it is possible and desirable to give it some rest, to minimize demands on it, and to help it recover and heal.

As you know, any movement you make uses up oxygen, which means that more oxygen is needed; since oxygen is carried in the blood, this means that increased circulation is required and, for that, more pumping work for the heart.

So, very early after a heart attack, you will be spoonfed and spongebathed to enable you to keep your own movements to a minimum.

But the restrictions won't last long. Once they would have. But it's now known that, everything considered—the heart and other parts of the body as well, including lungs and muscles—extended complete rest is not needed, nor is it good for the patient, who recovers more quickly with a gradual return to some activity.

Hence, as soon as the pain of the attack subsides, you should—and you probably will be encouraged to—start mild exercises. You should do them regularly and frequently—just moving your feet up and down, bending and unbending your knees, moving your arms.

The leg movements are to help avoid possible inflammation of the veins in the legs. The movements of your arms—lift them over your head every once in a while—may prevent pain about the shoulders.

You should breathe deeply, too, at regular intervals. And you should cough occasionally.

You will be assisted to a bedside commode for bowel movements.

THE HEART ATTACK

If your condition permits, you will soon be allowed to sit in a chair, where you should continue the exercises you have been doing in bed.

How Long Will I Stay in the Coronary Care Unit?

After about four days you may be transferred to a less intensive post-coronary care unit. But this will be done only when it is determined by the physician that you are out of immediate danger and no longer require continuous observation.

Your heart may still be monitored but your observation will be less intensive, because most of the difficulties associated with heart attacks that require immediate care occur within the first few hours or days.

How Long Before I Will Be Walking Around?

If your condition permits, your physician will have you increasingly active and you may find yourself walking around within two weeks.

You may feel unusually tired and unsteady on your feet. Many patients do. Don't let this worry you. It is a common occurrence after a heart attack. It may continue for several weeks after you return home.

Your heart has to heal completely and you will have to get back into condition. Then the tiredness will gradually subside as you recondition your body and your heart regains its strength.

What's Really the Purpose of All the Treatment Measures After an Attack?

There are actually several purposes. One is to help the healing of the heart. Another is to encourage new blood vessels to form—they're called collateral vessels—so that circulation is increased to both the damaged and the undamaged muscle area. And still another is to prevent complications.

How—and When—Does the Heart Heal?

You'll recall that the pain felt when the heart attack occurs is the ache in the damaged part of the heart—the area not getting blood because the particular vessel that feeds that area has been closed off.

For a time, the damaged muscle area struggles to keep going despite the lack of nourishment. And as long as the struggling goes on, there is pain.

But gradually the muscle fibers in the area either recover or no longer are able to contract. In the latter case, they swell, and they die. And at that point, the pain begins to diminish and then to disappear.

That's when healing starts.

The healing is much like the healing that takes place elsewhere in the body after damage. First, an army of white blood cells—leukocytes, they're called—is mustered. There is debris to be removed if healing is to take place; the dead muscle fibers have to go. White cells have the ability to engulf debris, in effect, wrapping themselves around the material.

It takes about a week, sometimes a little longer, for the debris removal to be completed. And during this time the patient experiences a little fever.

So the fever is a good sign—an indication that the leukocytes are at work, that the first stage of recovery has begun.

Where Do the New Blood Vessels Fit into the Picture?

The very minute a coronary vessel is choked off, there is a stimulus to the body to develop or open up new blood vessels. They may be small but they help to bring blood to the area around the damaged muscle—blood that helps in the healing process.

Another phenomenon often helps, too.

Before the heart attack, as atherosclerosis develops over an extended period, the slow narrowing may encourage the development of collateral vessels. If there has been time for a lot of collateral formation to have occurred before the blockage and heart attack occur, the collateral vessel pathways may help to save huge amounts of the heart muscle, very greatly limiting the area of damage, and so, of course, reducing the amount of healing that has to take place.

And still another phenomenon can help.

The coronary circulation is so designed that there are many interconnections between one coronary artery and another through many small branches and capillaries. Blood, of course, moves through the coronary arteries, as through all arteries, under pressure. When a coronary artery becomes blocked, pressure stops right there. Beyond the obstruction, there is no pressure at all.

That is good, because with normal pressure in unobstructed artery segments but no pressure beyond the blockage in the obstructed artery, there is a steep pressure gradient. And that tends to push some of the blood from good vessels through the interconnections into the obstructed artery at a point beyond the blockage.

So now, thanks to that detour, blood gets to the affected heart area through the original vessel feeding the area. That blood, too, helps in the healing.

Sometimes the detoured blood does even more. It is possible, especially when a heart attack is caused by an obstruction in a minor coronary branch, for the detoured blood to arrive quickly enough and in sufficient quantity at the small area of affected heart muscle to minimize the damage or even to assure that almost no lasting damage occurs.

This mechanism may account for the fact that a minor heart attack can occur with the victim remaining unaware and experiencing no discomfort.

How Does Healing Proceed After That?

When the debris has been cleared away, a scar begins to form in the damaged muscle area. It replaces the dead tissue. The scar is usually building up well within the first several weeks after the attack.

There are individual differences—individual healing rates

and, of course, differences from one person to another in the extent of injury. But usually within a month to six weeks the scar has become firm and tough.

How Long Will I Have to Stay in the Hospital?

Usually for two or three weeks.

What About the Possibility of Complications?

For many patients, recovery after a heart attack proceeds smoothly. Others experience complications. Major advances have been made in combatting and overcoming—and even preventing—serious complications.

We've already discussed one complication, arrhythmia—electrical failure. Serious heartbeat irregularities in the past have probably been responsible for most deaths after heart attacks. They still account for many, even most, deaths that occur out of the hospital.

But if you get to a hospital quickly—during an attack or shortly afterward—your chances not only of surviving a potentially deadly irregularity but of having it prevented from occurring are extremely high.

Another possible complication is shock.

What Is Shock? What Can Be Done for It?

Sometimes when there is injury to the heart muscle there is a reflex nerve action that causes arteries elsewhere in the body to open up wide.

When this happens, circulation in effect collapses. Blood "pools" in the wide-open arteries, blood pressure falls, the amount of circulating blood diminishes, the heart rate speeds up.

This is shock.

Shock can also occur after an injury such as a severe wound, a broken bone, massive bleeding, or extensive burns or upon dehydration (loss of body fluids because of extensive

The Heart Attack

vomiting, severe diarrhea, or extreme sweating). It may occur, too, during an allergic reaction to an insect sting or as the result of a severe infection or poisoning.

But no matter what the cause, shock must be properly treated to avoid further serious consequences. And in the hospital, of course, you can expect prompt and highly effective treatment.

Oxygen and other supportive measures may be used. Often, simple replacement of lost fluid by infusion will be effective, and one or more medications will be used to restore blood pressure and get circulation reestablished. Usually, an effective drug can produce a rise in blood pressure within a short time. Occasionally the intra-aortic balloon, mentioned earlier, may help.

Are There Any Other Possible Complications?

Pulmonary edema, or waterlogging of the lungs, sometimes may develop.

This, too, can be treated effectively. Oxygen can be administered, and digitalis may be used to strengthen the heart's pumping action, thus improving blood circulation so that fluids can be picked up from the lungs and carried by the blood to the kidneys to be eliminated in normal fashion. A diuretic—a drug designed to increase fluid elimination—may be used to avoid any recurrence of the edema.

We'll be discussing these and other medications in some detail in Chapter 7, so you will have full information about them.

Can Any Other Complication Develop?

Mild congestive heart failure is not uncommon in the first days after a heart attack.

Don't let the term alarm you. Failure doesn't mean that the heart is stopping. Rather, with the heart understandably stressed and weakened because of heart attack, the left ventricle, which pumps blood to the body, tends to contract a little less efficiently. Each time it contracts, it pumps some blood but some remains behind.

That leads to fluid congestion—some fluid accumulation in the lungs, tissue spaces, ankles, and perhaps abdomen.

Rarely is any intensive treatment needed. Salt tends to favor fluid accumulation, so its intake may be restricted. The use of a diuretic drug also helps. And as the heart regains its strength the congestive failure disappears.

Can There Be Emotional Complications? Do They Matter?

I'm glad you asked those questions.

There can be such complications. They do matter—and they can be handled and should be.

We touched a bit on how you're likely to feel and how anxiety is natural for anyone suffering a heart attack.

We should—and can—go further into emotional reactions than we did earlier.

What's Really Involved in the Emotional Reactions?

For one thing, the chances are that, like many—and perhaps most—other people, you have always thought of heart disease in terms of death—sudden death.

People who have had a heart attack may feel that, although they are progressing well, they are doomed—even if not immediately. They may be beset by the feeling that sooner or later, probably sooner, their heart will fail—for keeps.

But Isn't It True That There's Greater Risk Now?

Not by any means does the fact that you have had one heart attack make it inevitable that you will have another. It's simply impossible to make any 100 percent accurate forecasts about repeat attacks. They may come—but they don't inevitably have to come.

Incidentally, if there should be a repeat attack, it is not true that it must be more serious than the first. Nor is it true that a third attack, if it should ever come, must be fatal.

The Heart Attack

There are people who have survived second, third, fourth, and fifth heart attacks. The occurrence of several heart attacks in one person is not common, but survival is possible nonetheless.

If you're under competent medical care, and especially if you heed the warning of the first attack, you can do much to greatly minimize the chances of getting another attack.

We'll be discussing specifically how that can be done in Chapter 5.

Is Worry Over a Repeat the Only Emotional Reaction?

No. There is another common reaction.

A friend of mine, also a cardiologist, who himself experienced a very severe heart attack and recovered (recovered well enough to return to a most active medical practice and a distinguished career), expressed it well. He recalled the feeling, shortly after his attack, that there had been an insult to his ego because the attack had required "emotional and intellectual acknowledgment of vulnerability to death—an acknowledgment that plays havoc with the fantasy of immortality."

Most of us, probably all of us, for much of the time we go through life, have difficulty conceiving that we are mortal and will die. Oh, yes, we know we will—intellectually. But the gut feeling that we will is absent—until some day, somehow, we are shocked into an emotional acknowledgment.

This realization, for a time at least, can be a tough blow. But, however unnerving it may be, one does recover from it—and all the more quickly, if one faces up to it, realizes what has been happening, and acknowledges that the experience is a common one, coming to all of us, sometimes as a result of a heart attack, sometimes as a result of another illness or event.

How Do Heart Attack Victims Usually React Emotionally?

Some become excessively anxious. They are almost overpoweringly worried about their hearts. They have difficulty sleeping. Their state of mind is almost wholly one of apprehension. Anyone seeing them—certainly the physician attending them—can't help but be aware of their state of mind.

Some are just as anxious but they don't show it. They try to bury the anxiety. And they may make such great efforts to keep the anxiety buried that they themselves are not acutely aware of it. They work at controlling themselves, at staying calm, at following medical orders meticulously.

There are still others who react with a complete denial of anxiety. They act as though they have not had an attack. After they recover, they make a point of being vigorous, excessively vigorous. They may undertake a superman's work or sports, expending energy far greater than any normally healthy person would or than they would have before their attack. They are using a mental mechanism which says no to any facts that might produce anxiety, denies their very existence.

Finally, there are those who go into depression.

Depressed feelings—blue feelings—are normal after a heart attack. Those feelings stem from a loss, as depressed feelings often do. It's normal to feel depressed after the loss of a loved one, the loss of a job, a financial loss, or almost any other kind of loss that has meaning for the individual.

With a heart attack, of course, there is a series of losses—the loss of invulnerability to mortality, for one, and the loss of the feeling of being basically healthy. Suddenly, now, with the heart attack, one may see oneself as a total invalid.

But as soon as one's strength is regained, confidence returns, and with it the depression should depart.

That's the normal course for post-heart-attack depression.

But some who have heart attacks don't follow that pattern. Their depression is severe, and it goes on and on. They become apathetic. They withdraw. They feel worthless. They despair. They may turn on friends. They may even withdraw from loved ones. They retreat into themselves. They become uncommunicative.

What Can Be Done for Such Anxious or Depressed Patients?

I mention these varying reactions with the hope that if you are ever a heart attack victim you may better identify what your reactions are.

Half the battle is in recognizing what is a normal, healthy reaction and what is not. If it is normal and healthy, it will be relatively brief—a matter of days, perhaps weeks. And if you understand the nature of your anxiety or depression, that's to the good. You will be helped by the understanding, and the period of upset is likely to be abbreviated. Talking about your feelings could help greatly too.

If your reaction diverges from the normal, it's a help to recognize that it is diverging—and a help also to realize that you can, in fact, be helped. Your physician may be able to be of great help to you, for your emotional trauma as well as the physical. Or your physician may advise—even while you are still in the hospital or perhaps soon afterward—that you get psychiatric help, which need not be a long-drawn-out process. There are techniques for dealing with crisis situations—and yours may be a kind of crisis that needs and can have a quick resolution. The resolution will very materially aid your recovery and your return to a full life.

Is All the Emotional Upset Concentrated in the Period Immediately After the Heart Attack?

To a large extent, it is likely to be.

But you may have some ups and downs of feelings later on—and that will be natural.

There may be times when you feel irritable or impatient. It's understandable that even though you may make fast progress in recovery you may at times wish it were faster, and so, briefly, you become a little irritated or depressed.

But there will be times, too, when you make what seem to be sudden, significant gains—finding yourself able perhaps to do easily one day what was more difficult the last time you tried it. At those times, you may feel euphoric—very, very elated.

If you swing a bit back and forth, feeling very satisfied some of the time and less so at other times, that's not unusual or abnormal. It happens in other aspects of life too.

It's only when—and this is not inevitable at all—you experience an extended period of discouragement or depression or anxiety that you may neep help. At that point, don't delay in talking things over with your physician. He or she very definitely can help.

4

Afterward

You've had a heart attack. What can you expect to happen in the days, weeks, months, even years, ahead? What will be done for you—and why? What will you be doing for yourself—and why? How soon can you become active—to what extent? When can you return to work and to other activities?

When the Heart Heals, Does It, in Effect, Become Whole Again?

In one sense, no. The dead area of heart muscle cannot be restored and is replaced by scar tissue.

But that need not matter significantly. Unless too much heart muscle has been destroyed in the attack, the remaining healthy heart muscle, once the healing process is complete, can usually provide satisfactory pumping rhythm and force. After a heart attack, in fact, some patients who suffered before from angina are completely freed of the chest pain.

How Is It Possible to Be Angina-Free Afterward?

This may happen if the impaired heart muscle area—which caused the angina in the first place, due to insufficient blood and oxygen supply—is replaced by scar tissue. Scar tissue does not require oxygen and does not cause pain.

Why Do I Feel So Weak and Tired?

After a heart attack many patients feel very weak and tired. You should not be alarmed about these feelings for they are common in these circumstances.

Not long after an attack you may be encouraged to become somewhat active. Still, the activity necessarily will be limited in order to aid healing. With relative inactivity, even a healthy person loses much energy, feels more tired and weak, until he gets back into shape.

Weakness is not a sign of complication, nor does it mean that your heart condition is getting worse again. Rather, it is an expected part of your recovery. The weakness will begin to pass as you gradually increase your activity and regain strength and endurance.

How Soon Can I Become Active?

If your heart attack was uncomplicated—that is, without shock, heart failure, or dangerous abnormal rhythms—you may be able to resume some activities quite early.

Usually, your physician will prescribe leg, arm, and breathing exercises while you are in the hospital. The degree of activity permitted will gradually increase.

At first, you may use the commode with assistance. Later you may walk to the bathroom. You may sit up in a chair and feed and shave yourself. You can comb or set your hair and wash yourself.

Prior to discharge from the hospital, you will be allowed to walk up and down the corridor. Of course, if any of this causes you chest discomfort, abnormal heart-rate changes, short-windedness, blood-pressure elevation or rhythm disturbance, the activity should be halted.

If Chest Pain Returns, Does It Mean I'm Having Another Heart Attack?

Not necessarily. If the pain is triggered by physical effort or emotional upset, is short-lasting, and responds to nitroglycerin, it is only caused by angina. However, if it persists and is not relieved by nitroglycerin, then one possibility is that it represents an extension of the previous heart attack.

Another possibility is that chest-wall and/or shoulder pain may occur intermittently in the early weeks after a heart attack, becoming worse when you move the affected part of the body. This is a localized condition that is neither angina nor heart attack. It will not respond to nitroglycerin but often does respond to anti-inflammatory agents such as aspirin, indomethacin, or cortisone.

Also, occasionally, a few weeks after a heart attack, a patient may become feverish and experience chest pains while inhaling. Such pain, which may last for days, usually responds to drugs that reduce inflammation. It is due to a relatively harmless, usually self-limited, sometimes recurrent inflammation of the outer lining of the heart (the pericardium) caused by the heart attack. It is called *Dressler's syndrome* or *postmyocardial infarction syndrome.*

Pain that is severe, persistent, or recurrent is an indication that you should consult your physician.

What Will Happen After I Leave the Hospital?

Your physician will have advice and a plan for recovery that you should follow faithfully. The instructions may vary according to your particular situation and your condition upon discharge from the hospital.

Usually, it is a good idea to continue for about two weeks at home the same activities you were allowed in the hospital. Then, gradually, according to your physician's instructions, you can increase your activities and add new ones over the several months you will need to recover fully from a heart attack.

How Soon Before I Can Engage in More Vigorous Activities?

After an uncomplicated heart attack, you should wait about four weeks to two months before attempting such more-vigorous activities as brisk walking and light calisthenics. And then, before you begin, you should have a careful checkup by your physician.

It isn't often necessary, but under certain circumstances your physician may want to give you a stress test (see page 145) which can provide valuable information on how much exercise you can do and how long you should do it.

Even if you have angina after a heart attack and the angina has remained stable for several months, you can start exercising if the exercise causes no distress. A program of carefully supervised exercise may sometimes even reduce the angina. Your local heart association may sponsor such exercise programs and you can participate if your physician approves.

Why Is Exercise So Beneficial?

Exercise can increase your sense of well-being and decrease the extreme fatigue experienced after a heart attack.

When you are in good physical condition, exercise and other physical exertion require less heart effort—the heart rate increases less and blood pressure rises less—than when you are out of shape. In good condition, you use less oxygen for any given activity and are able to do more physical work. Exercise may also reduce blood fat levels.

For these reasons, regular exercise should be part of everyone's life.

After a heart attack a well-planned program of gradually increasing activity can go far toward making you feel well again and improving the quality of your life. It may even prolong life, but there is no scientific proof of this yet.

In time, such exercise may decrease the frequency and severity of angina by promoting better utilization of oxygen and a lesser increase of heart rate and blood pressure during activity.

Can I Climb Stairs?

Usually yes, after an uncomplicated heart attack—and, often, even if you have angina. And you can usually do so, slowly,

Afterward

resting every few steps if necessary, as soon as you get home from the hospital.

But do not climb steps right after a meal.

Again, for emphasis, climb slowly and stop and rest if you get chest pains, become unusually short of breath, or feel your heart beating irregularly or too fast.

Gradually you may find that you are able to climb more rapidly and with fewer or no rest stops.

If the effort of climbing still bothers you, you may find it necessary to climb only when it is unavoidable. If you experience chest pains while climbing, your physician may suggest that you place a nitroglycerin tablet under your tongue two minutes before.

If you suddenly experience discomfort where none had existed before, you should promptly report this to your physician. A slight change in your medication may bring improvement.

In rare cases, it is advisable to avoid all stair climbing. This sometimes may require installation of a stair elevator.

How Soon After the Heart Attack Can I Shower, Bathe, and Swim?

If you've had an uncomplicated attack, you can usually shower or bathe several weeks afterward. Of course, before that, even in the hospital, you can give yourself sponge baths.

Avoid water that is too hot or too cold, since extremes of temperature may disturb your heart rhythm or lead to chest discomfort. Use lukewarm water only—water not very different in temperature from that of your body.

The first few times you shower or bathe, you should have assistance. If self-bathing leads to any chest discomfort, you should stop.

On the other hand, it's usually advisable to postpone swimming for three or four months after an attack. Then, to begin with, you would be well-advised to do your swimming in the presence of a lifeguard, close to land or to the edge of the pool. The water should not be very cold or hot. Don't jump in;

enter the water gradually. Don't swim after meals. Start out swimming short distances and, if there are no difficulties, you can gradually increase the distances.

Is It All Right to Exercise or Work After Meals?

No!

After a meal, blood is needed by the organs that digest your food. The blood vessels supplying your stomach and intestines dilate and some of the blood that otherwise would be available to supply your heart muscle goes to the digestive system.

With work or exercise, the heart muscle needs more oxygen and therefore more blood. It's a strain on even the normal cardiovascular system to provide the additional blood for the heart muscle at the same time it is meeting the demand of stomach and intestinal tract for more blood.

It's likely to be all the more of a strain or even an impossibility when the cardiovascular system is not entirely normal. That is why many heart patients cannot work or even walk after meals without chest discomfort, even though they may have no such discomfort before meals.

Heart patients should rest in a comfortable chair for half an hour to an hour after each meal. Also, your physician may suggest that you eat smaller meals to make digestion easier.

What About Jogging?

It has become a popular form of exercise for cardiac patients, but you should try jogging only under the close supervision of a physician. After it is clear that you can maintain an exercise routine and are properly conditioned for it, then you may carry it out on your own with your physician's knowledge and approval, and the routine may include jogging if done noncompetitively.

A brisk walk before dinner, gradually increasing its tempo and distance, is probably as good a way, especially early on, to get into shape as jogging. Your physician may advise certain traditional exercises. Follow all instructions, since your physician knows *your* body and *your* heart.

When Can I Go Back to Work?

It's usually advisable to wait for about two months until your heart muscle is adequately healed.

Can I Return to the Same Job?

Chances are good that you can.

As a rule, it's best that you go back to the job you had before the heart attack if possible. By doing so, you return to a known situation and to friends on the job. This may avoid for you a great deal of anxiety that frequently arises in connection with a new job.

At some point, however, you should discuss the daily routine of your job with your physician. Many jobs demand only minimal physical effort, with much of the heavy work being performed by machines. It is possible that there are occasional tasks in your work that require physical strain, and these should be avoided. Frequently, this can be arranged after a discussion of your condition with the plant physician, employer, union representative, or fellow workers.

Actually, recently made measurements have been showing just how low an expenditure of physical energy is required by many factory, white-collar, and service jobs. The Scientific Council on Rehabilitation has measured energy costs in METS. A MET represents the amount of oxygen a person consumes at rest. That amounts to 3.5 milliliters—or about 3½ thousandths of a quart—of oxygen per minute for each kilogram (2.2 pounds) of body weight.

When you do desk work, the energy cost is 1½ to 2 METS—at most, a doubling of the energy cost at rest. For radio-TV repair, the expenditure is 2 to 3 METS; for bricklaying, plastering, or machine assembly, 3 to 4 METS; for painting, 4 to 5; and for shoveling, depending on the load, 6 to 10 METS.

Stress tests (see page 145) can determine how much work you can perform comfortably, without any undue elevation of your heart rate and blood pressure. The amount of energy expenditure required at your job may have already been determined or may be estimated. And based on the amount of energy you can expend without undue symptoms, your physician can determine whether you can return to your old job or whether your job has to be modified or completely changed.

If it should turn out that your old job is unsafe for you, you should seriously consider changing jobs. Your physician and local rehabilitation center may be able to help you with the problem.

There are certain jobs for which a heart condition will disqualify you. For example, you will not qualify to be an airline pilot, bus driver, locomotive engineer, or an astronaut.

The likelihood that you will have to stop working entirely is very small. If this should be the case and you are still under age sixty-five, you may still be eligible for Social Security payments. You may also be eligible for disability insurance compensation from your place of work. If you are a veteran, you may be able to qualify for a veteran's disability pension.

If you have more than one job, there is strong medical reason for giving up the second job. It is far better to make your economic needs more modest and live on less money for a longer time than to earn for a short time the higher income of two jobs.

May I Continue to Work If I Have Angina?

Very likely, yes.

However, it is best that you avoid situations of severe physical or emotional strain. Depending upon the nature of your job, it is possible that you may have to work, at least for a time, at a slower pace and take periodic rests.

By all means, don't just give up work if you have angina and assume that work is impossible. Rather, consult your physician about your work.

Afterward

Nitroglycerin is an important drug for you if you have angina, and it may sometimes be valuable on the job. Should there be an activity that, in your experience, tends to cause you chest discomfort, it may be advisable, if your physician agrees, to place a nitroglycerin tablet under your tongue before commencing such an activity if it cannot be avoided.

If, despite such a precaution, discomfort occurs, the activity should be discontinued temporarily and you should place one, and if necessary another, nitroglycerin tablet under your tongue until the discomfort subsides, after which you can try to resume your work.

Your work need not increase the number of your angina attacks. It's quite possible that there will be no increase in angina attacks even without any adjustments in your job. And, frequently, if a readjustment is needed, your employer will help make it. You should feel free to ask your physician to contact your employer and give him full information about your condition.

Please note this: There are many myths about heart disease. Your employer may not have had occasion to learn the truth about it. And your physician's explanation to him can often do much to ease the way for you.

Can I Resume Housework After Recovering from a Heart Attack?

Yes, you can. But wait seven or eight weeks before doing so. Then, if your physician finds you well enough and if your heart attack was uncomplicated, it is perfectly all right.

But start slowly, avoid sudden strains, and do not work when you are upset. Should you get angina, sit down for a while and take a nitroglycerin tablet.

Are There Household Activities I Should Avoid?

Some heavy activities should be avoided, since they frequently trigger angina: scrubbing floors, turning mattresses, vacuuming, carrying heavy bundles, toting laundry baskets, raking leaves, cutting grass, and shoveling snow.

Your family should be informed that it is medically inadvisable for you to perform such tasks. Perhaps other members of the family can do them.

Do not work for half an hour to an hour after a meal.

If your house has more than one floor, do the work on one floor before going on to the next, so that you will not have to run up and down stairs frequently. Take your time, and take frequent rests. Don't be compulsive about keeping your home or apartment immaculate.

Work outdoors only when the temperature is moderate. If it is very cold or very hot, you are better off remaining indoors with heat or air-conditioning until the outdoor temperature becomes milder. Light gardening, if you like it, is a fine activity.

In general, housework, like exercise or work at a job in business or industry, is fine if done at an easy pace without anxiety and with avoidance of any specific activities that cause you extreme stress or strain.

Is There a Particular Kind of Muscular Activity I Should Avoid?

Yes, the kind called isometric.

In isometric activity, you apply a muscle with great force to push or pull against an immovable object such as a wall, or you pit the muscle against the opposition of another muscle.

Such isometric activity is frequently used in exercises to make bulging muscles such as the biceps and triceps in the arms. And, indeed, isometric workouts can produce big "beach boy"-type muscles but contribute nothing to building heart muscle tone and endurance. For the latter, dynamic activities—such as walking, jogging, swimming, bicycling, and other efforts in which large groups of muscles participate and for longer periods—are needed.

Isometric activity is also involved in certain types of work such as lifting heavy objects, opening stuck windows, pushing or pulling a stalled car, turning a very tight crank.

Isometric work and exercise should be avoided by anyone with a heart condition, because such activity produces sudden

AFTERWARD

increases in heart rate and blood pressure. Isometric activity can, in fact, cause angina and may even precipitate a heart attack or stroke in someone with a heart problem. Lord Moran, physician to Winston Churchill, has reported on how Churchill suffered an episode of coronary insufficiency after straining to open a White House window during a 1941 visit to Washington.

Are There Particular Sports and Other Activities to Be Wary Of?

Activities in which any sort of great effort is required or in which the effort is not easy and steady are not recommended. These would include such games as tennis, football, soccer, and even badminton or table tennis.

In general, any competitive sport should be avoided if it is played to win rather than for the fun of it. Bowling and golf are good exercises but, if played to win, to compete, to excel, they may overtax you and be bad for you. Emotional tension adds to the physical strain of any game or sport.

Doing work with your arms over your head, as in painting, for example, may also cause distress, especially if done in a hurry.

Of course, as mentioned earlier, all work should be avoided immediately after meals and in extremes of hot, humid, or cold weather, and it is wise to avoid if possible such chores as raking leaves, cutting grass, shoveling snow, vacuuming, turning mattresses, and carrying heavy bundles.

Finally, if in doubt about a particular kind of work or exercise that is important to you, feel free to consult your physician. In general, steady and easy-does-it work is best for you—and activities that are sudden, excessively strenuous, uneven, or competitive are best avoided.

If I Experience Chest Discomfort, Extreme Short-windedness, or Heart Rhythm Disturbances While Exercising, Should I Continue in the Hope That They May Disappear?

No, you should stop exercising immediately, and take a nitroglycerin tablet. If the symptoms do not disappear in a short time after taking two additional nitroglycerin tablets, if necessary, two to three minutes apart, you should be taken to the emergency room of a hospital or call an ambulance. If the pain or discomfort persists, you may be having a heart attack.

After such an incident, your physician may advise you to hold off exercising for a while longer. When you resume, he or she may advise a slower start. Medication may be prescribed to improve the performance of your heart and your physician may recommend that in the future you take a nitroglycerin tablet before beginning exercise.

What About Sexual Activity After a Heart Attack?

This question often worries patients. It need not worry you.

Like other exercise, sexual activity is something that should be resumed slowly, usually about seven or eight weeks after the attack. The exact time depends upon the severity of the attack, your condition on discharge from the hospital, and the rapidity of your recovery afterward.

Before discharge, you and your spouse should discuss this question with your physician.

At the beginning, intercourse should be as calm and restful as possible. Take it easy; don't work too hard; don't feel a need to prove something to your spouse.

You may want to lie on your back with your spouse on top. And, at first, it may be wise to have your partner undertake most of the activity.

There is no reason to fear the sex act. The energy expended is no more than it would take for you to climb two flights of stairs or to walk a city block briskly. Intercourse does increase blood pressure, pulse rate, and the work of the heart, but by seven or eight weeks after an attack most patients can easily tolerate this. Nor is there any reason whatever to fear having an orgasm.

You should wait at least two hours after a meal before any sexual activity. Your partner, initially, should not insist on having an orgasm if that requires great physical effort on your part.

Afterward

You may find yourself having to discuss things that could have been taken for granted before your heart attack.

Extramarital sex has been found to cause anxiety, guilt, and fear of detection. Consequently, it is often associated with cardiac complications.

Sexual abstinence may not be a good idea since sexual fantasies may cause strain.

Have no doubt that, given a little time, you will be able to perform the sex act adequately. Do not hesitate to tell your partner of your problems and wishes.

A woman, after a heart attack, should avoid pregnancy—but by means other than the use of birth control pills.

In general, if you take it slow and easy at the beginning, without feeling a need to prove anything to your partner or yourself, and if you refuse to worry about it, sex will take care of itself.

What Should I Do If I Experience Angina or Become Extremely Short of Breath During Intercourse?

It is wise to discontinue and consult your physician before attempting sexual activity again.

Usually, your physician will be able to completely relieve any difficulties by prescribing proper medication. A long-acting form of nitroglycerin may be prescribed to be taken fifteen minutes before the sex act, combined with a regular nitroglycerin tablet to be used about two minutes before. Should intercourse be prolonged beyond fifteen minutes, the regular tablet can be taken again.

Sometimes, other drugs are necessary. Propranolol can be useful since it decreases the heart rate and oxygen needs of the heart.

If there is extreme shortness of breath, particularly if that is associated with wheezing, digitalis may be used to increase the heart's strength and capacity for pumping and a diuretic may be employed to increase fluid outflow via the urine so as to overcome congestion.

An episode of discomfort during sexual activity does not mean that you must experience such discomfort every time you engage in sex. Nor does it mean that you are likely to provoke a heart attack with sex. The appropriate medications can make sexual activity safe and painless.

You should feel free to discuss any difficulties with intercourse not only with your physician but with your sex partner as well. The partner's understanding and supporting and loving attitude can do much to alleviate any anxieties you may have.

Your partner should feel free to touch, embrace, and fondle you, to initiate lovemaking, and, as suggested earlier, to take a more active part in foreplay than before cardiac difficulties occurred.

May I Drive After a Heart Attack?

If you have to drive in heavy traffic or in very cold or very hot, humid weather, or for long distances, your heart could be taxed. Otherwise, you can probably start driving in ten to twelve weeks. If you must drive a car or truck without power steering, you should probably wait at least twelve weeks after your attack.

Tests have established that after a heart attack the heart may be susceptible to rhythm disturbances during driving. But this danger greatly decreases as time goes on.

In the final analysis, whether and at what point you should drive depends upon your individual rate of recovery, the type of driving, and the advice of your physician.

May I Travel?

Yes, but there are some precautions that are good to keep in mind.

Riding as a passenger can be done safely earlier than driving, probably within five to six weeks after an uncomplicated attack.

If you travel for a long distance in a car, the car should be stopped frequently so that you can get out and exercise your legs by walking around. This will help to prevent blood clots in your legs. It might well be added here that this practice is just as advisable for people who have no heart problem.

By all means, avoid the stress of rushing to get anywhere. If you are traveling for business, leave a little early so you can travel without haste. And if you are traveling on vacation, remember that a cardinal value of a vacation should be the relaxation it affords.

You should assure yourself opportunity for ample rest at night. You can do this and avoid needless anxiety by phoning ahead for reservations.

It is generally a bad idea to travel in a hot car or public conveyance in hot weather. It might be advisable, if your car does not already have an air conditioner, to install one and where possible to find public conveyances that are air-conditioned. Be sure, too, that the room in which you stay is air-conditioned.

In trains, buses, or airplanes make yourself comfortable and make a practice of getting up every hour or so to stretch your legs and walk around a bit—again to help avoid blood clotting in the legs.

Is Plane Travel Safe?

There should be no difficulty in traveling by plane. Commercial airliners are pressurized above a level of 5,000 feet. Since you will not be engaged in any physical effort while on the plane, this altitude is usually easily tolerated. If flying makes you anxious, it is a good idea to take a mild sedative before you get on the plane. And of course you should carry your medications with you at all times, no matter where or how you travel.

If you have any difficulty breathing or feel otherwise uncomfortable, don't hesitate to tell a stewardess about it. Oxygen is readily available at every seat.

Are There Any Other Precautions I Should Take in Traveling?

Under no circumstances should you carry anything much heavier than a briefcase. There usually are people available to carry your luggage. But if, for some reason, there should not be, you should not feel embarrassed to ask train or plane personnel for help.

Before leaving on an extended trip, it is a good idea to get a report from your physician describing your condition and a copy of your latest electrocardiogram. It's advisable to determine the location and phone number of the hospital nearest to where you will be vacationing. If you are going to a foreign country, you should obtain a list of English-speaking physicians from the International Association for Medical Assistance to Travelers.

Following these simple rules will pay off if an emergency should occur.

Is It Safe for Me to Take a Vacation After a Heart Attack?

Yes, it is safe. But you should not try to do so until three to six months have elapsed since the attack. After the initial healing has taken place, it is perfectly safe to travel and have fun. If you have any questions at all about taking a vacation, you can and should get the advice of your physician.

You will have to take the same precautions during your vacation as you do during your everyday life at home. A vacation is a time to relax, enjoy yourself, and be carefree, but it is not a time to take unwise chances.

You may find a cruise very relaxing, but you should avoid eating large meals, rich food, or drinking alcohol. Discuss your diet with the steward. Be sure to take rest periods and don't stay up too late for parties.

If the ship makes stops for sightseeing, inquire beforehand about the amount of walking involved. You should avoid situations where you will have to walk up hills, and it is bad to go sightseeing immediately after eating.

Be sure to take a sufficient amount of your medication with you. As a precaution, add a couple of weeks of extra medication supplies. It is better to have some excess than to run short.

Avoid vacations in climates of extreme heat or cold, and choose a site that is less than 3,000 feet above sea level. If there are extreme temperatures during part of the day, you should avoid them by "staying put" in comfort, reading, relaxing, perhaps taking a "siesta."

If you find the sightseeing becoming too strenuous, you should not hesitate to remain on the sightseeing bus, train, or boat.

Remember: relaxation, leisure, and fun within the limits prescribed by your physician make sense. Leave your cares behind you and bon voyage!

May I Drink Alcoholic Beverages?

There is little doubt that heavy drinking is bad for your heart, as well as for most of your body. Alcoholics may develop beriberi heart disease as the result of vitamin B deficiency. Or they may experience the heart disease known as alcoholic myocardiopathy, resulting from the toxic effects of excessive alcohol on the heart muscle. It's urgent for such patients to stop all drinking immediately and have treatment that includes proper nutrition, medication, and rest.

What about light drinking? It depends on what you mean by "light." It might be a good idea for you to keep a log for a few weeks and measure your actual intake of alcohol, rather than depend on what you *think* you drink.

Physicians still differ in their conclusions about light drinking for heart patients. There has been a general feeling that a drink may not hurt and may actually help prevent angina. But in the past few years some cardiologists have come to believe that alcohol, even in small quantities, is bad for the heart.

The new belief stems from laboratory studies indicating that as little as two ounces of alcohol a day may increase the damage to an already damaged heart and greatly decrease the heart's pumping efficiency.

Alcohol in such amounts may also disturb heart rhythm, perhaps producing extra beats or irregular beats (atrial fibrillation). Such abnormal rhythms, or arrhythmias, can cause discomfort and anxiety and may dangerously decrease the efficiency of the heart.

Relatively small amounts of alcohol also increase the level

of fats (triglycerides) in the blood and may also increase blood pressure.

Given this knowledge, it would seem prudent to allow oneself each day no more than one cocktail or one glass of wine or beer. Don't have more than one drink—and avoid even the one if it causes any disturbance of your heart rhythm.

May I Go to Parties, Dance, Resume a Social Life After Recovering from a Heart Attack?

A heart attack need not, and should not, make you a social invalid any more than it should make you a physical invalid for the rest of your life.

On the contrary, it is good not to dwell on your heart problem and to live as normally as possible, providing you follow the guidelines outlined for you by your physician.

Yes, you can go to parties and give them, and dance, and resume your social life, hobbies, and other activities, once your physician finds you have sufficiently recovered from your illness.

Your own reactions will help guide you, too. If, in the beginning, you come home from work feeling fatigued, it's wise to relax, have dinner, and go to bed early. As you become accustomed again to work, fatigue is likely to diminish and finally disappear. And when you can tolerate a day's work and an evening of social activity, there is no reason why you shouldn't enjoy doing so and, in fact, benefit from the camaraderie and cheer of friends.

Remember, however, that adequate rest is important. Leave parties early; don't be the last to leave. Don't attend parties every night and, if you dance, sit out every other dance if you begin to tire.

Don't dance immediately after a meal; allow at least a two-hour interval. Don't eat excessively at a party; eat only the main course, not a full-course meal. At most, have one drink—and not even that if you have found that heartbeat irregularity or chest discomfort result from it.

AFTERWARD

Can I Smoke?

If you do, you are foolish.

As the message on every pack of cigarettes indicates, "The Surgeon General has determined that smoking is hazardous to your health."

And if you have had a heart attack or suffer from angina, smoking is not just hazardous but suicidal.

Specifically—

Cigarettes, and to a lesser degree, cigars and pipes, are harmful to your lungs. Not only can they cause lung cancer, but they can foster obstructive lung disease or emphysema as well. By dilating the small air sacs in the lungs, they restrict the exchange of oxygen and carbon dioxide. This effect on your lungs is dangerous for your heart. Anything that inhibits oxygen supply to the heart muscle might aggravate an existing heart condition or even cause heart disease.

The nicotine in tobacco constricts blood vessels, thus interfering with normal blood flow. This adds to the work burden of the heart and leads to weakening of the heart muscle. Nicotine also increases the level in the blood of certain chemical substances, called catecholamines, which make the heart beat faster and often irregularly. Nicotine is a potent drug with potentially serious effects on your heart, especially when you have a heart problem.

Smoking increases the lipid, or fat, levels in your blood and also increases the stickiness of the blood platelets, increasing the probability that blood clots will form in the arteries, with a serious threat to life.

The carbon monoxide in smoke reaches the blood and decreases the ability of blood cells to carry oxygen, reducing the supply available to the heart.

In a patient with other risk factors (Chapter 5), smoking may greatly increase the likelihood of a heart attack at an early age, as well as increase the likelihood of a repeat after a first attack.

It is notable that, with the increase of smoking among women, young women who in the past did not ordinarily suffer from coronary heart disease today are experiencing an increased incidence of the disease. There is a possibility, too, that the use of the birth control pill will increase the likelihood of the ill effect of smoking in some women.

To succeed in giving up smoking requires adequate motivation and, everything considered, you certainly should have that. When you jeopardize your life, you do more, jeopardizing your family's welfare. Your smoking sets a bad example for your children. It also exposes your family to smoke itself, and breathing smoke-filled air can be hazardous.

Giving up smoking "cold turkey" is often the best way to stop. You may find a smoking clinic helpful. The first few weeks of giving up such a long-entrenched habit will very probably be difficult, with the difficulty diminishing markedly after that. Your physician may prescribe a mild sedative for the initial period of difficulty.

When you succeed in stopping smoking, you will be amazed at how much better you will feel. If you're experiencing any angina, there is likely to be less of it. Your head will be clearer, your senses of taste and smell enhanced, your breathing will be more natural and easy, you will be less tired—and these are only a few of the rewards of your victory over the addiction.

It is preferable that you stop smoking altogether. If you are truly unable to stop, however, the less you smoke the better. Pipe and cigar smoking are probably less harmful than cigarette smoking.

Should I Change My Diet?

That depends upon what your diet was prior to your heart attack or angina. If it was leading to excessive weight or was high in saturated fats and cholesterol, or both, you should definitely make changes.

Eat small meals, never heavy, full-course ones. Eat less, more often. Restrict salt intake, especially if you have high blood pressure or congestive heart failure. Avoid excessive sugar, too. Substitutes for sweets and salt can be used in moderation.

Pastry, candy, ice cream, cookies, doughnuts, pies, and

other sweets should be avoided, except as an occasional treat, not only because of sugar content but also because they have a high content of fat (triglyceride).

Avoid processed meats, sausages, hot dogs, bologna, and salami, all of which contain much fat and salt.

Reduce your intake of foods high in cholesterol, such as egg yolks. Reduce your intake of saturated fats: trim fat from your meat, avoid bacon, liver and other organ meats, whole milk, cream, butter, margarines containing saturated fats, lard, whipped cream.

Avoid prepared sauces such as ketchup, steak sauce, mustard and mayonnaise, since they contain a lot of salt.

You should eat lean meats, fish, and fowl without the skin, in moderate quantities. Use unsaturated oils such as corn and safflower oil. Eat vegetables, fruits, and salads.

Bread is permissible but should be eaten sparingly, particularly if you are overweight. Use skim milk, cottage cheese, nonfat yogurt, and other low-fat dairy products.

For more detailed information and for interesting recipes, consult a low-cholesterol cookbook such as those made available by the American Heart Association or by the U.S. Department of Health, Education, and Welfare, Public Health Service, 333 Independence Avenue SW, Washington, D.C. 20201.

After a Heart Attack, Am I Likely to Suffer Another?

Compared to people who have had no heart attack, the risk is increased—but only slightly.

No one can predict whether a person will have a repeat attack. But it is definitely a fact that a second attack is not inevitable.

Nor is it true, as so commonly believed, that a second attack, if it should occur, is more serious than the first and that a third attack is fatal. Second and third attacks can just as well be minor as major, and many patients have recovered from as many as half a dozen attacks.

Actually, if you are under the care of a competent physician and have heeded the warning of the first attack, chances of getting another heart attack may be markedly decreased. I have a great number of patients living productive and enjoyable lives many years after the first heart attack. So has every physician. Think of Presidents Eisenhower and Johnson who lived long after their first heart attacks, despite the strenuous, stressful work of the presidency.

The important thing is to follow competent medical advice. With today's medical insights into the causes of coronary heart disease and heart attack, and with the medical tools already available and the new ones constantly being researched and developed, the odds are that you will live a rewarding and productive life for many years to come. You will find more detailed information and guidelines on this in Chapter 5.

5

Decreasing the Risks of Occurrence and Recurrence

Happily, after having had a heart attack, you are recovering or have recovered. Can you avoid another? Or, not yet having had an attack, you are concerned—perhaps because you have angina or because of family history of attacks or for other reasons—that you may be on the way to having one. Can you avoid a first occurrence?

If I've Had a Heart Attack, Am I More Likely to Suffer Another Than If I Haven't Had One?

Yes. Statistics indicate that—overall—people who have had one "coronary" have a slightly increased chance of having a second, as compared with those who have never had one. But it's not true that once you have a heart attack you will inevitably have another.

If you've had an attack, you may well considerably reduce the chances of having another, possibly even to well below those of many who have never had an attack or an indication of heart trouble. Why? Because, more immediately than they, you have an interest in the disease, the factors involved in producing it, and what can be done to minimize or eliminate them.

What Are My Chances of Having a Heart Attack If I Have Angina?

It is far from inevitable, too, that you will have a first or a repeat heart attack if you have angina.

Are My Chances of an Attack, Original or Repeat, Greater If I Belong to Some Particular Category of People?

A heart attack may occur to anyone, at any age, of any race or nationality, and of either sex. But there is some difference in the likelihood depending on the group to which one belongs.

Statistics show, for example, that white American men—as a group—have the greatest chance of suffering heart attacks (often surprisingly early in life, occasionally in the twenties and thirties) and that their risk increases with age.

It's also a statistical fact that women are less likely than men to suffer heart attacks during the years when they are still capable of bearing children. But advancing age eliminates what seems to be a "hormonal shield" that they have.

We also know that some women who are smokers or who use oral contraceptives have a greater risk than other women who do not use them.

But not all white males, young or old, have heart attacks. Nor are all young women protected, with or without the use of cigarettes or of oral contraceptives. Nor do all who use the Pill or smoke have heart attacks.

Obviously, other factors are involved.

To take nationality as another example—in the United States and certain other countries, such as Finland, the number of heart attacks is very high. On the other hand, in some countries—such as Japan—heart attacks are relatively rare. But when Japanese move to the United States there is a decided change. First- and second-generation Japanese-Americans have heart attack rates approximating those of Americans. This suggests that environmental and cultural factors have a greater influence than nationality or racial inheritance in setting the stage for heart disease.

It's important not to leap to any conclusion about your risk just because you belong to some particular group. What is true for the group overall may not be true for a particular individual within the group.

What matters is why certain groups have a higher risk while others have a lower risk. What are the factors that in-

DECREASING THE RISKS OF OCCURRENCE AND RECURRENCE 83

crease risk? And can individuals surmount those factors, minimize their influence, and escape being a statistic?

We have been learning a good deal—more and more every year—about those risk factors and what can be done about them.

What Are the Risk Factors?

They include a family history of heart attacks at an early age, high blood pressure, high blood lipid (fat) levels (cholesterol and possibly triglycerides), smoking, diabetes, a certain type of personality (overly ambitious, competitive, aggressive, impatient, creating too many deadlines). Overweight, physical inactivity, stress, and high uric-acid levels are also suspected to be risk factors.

Risk factors are cumulative; that is, the more risk factors you have, the more likely you are to have coronary heart disease—angina, an original heart attack, and repeat heart attacks.

Moreover—and this is also quite significant—many risk factors interact. Are you overweight, for example? It may be due in part to your diet and in part to physical inactivity. Diabetes, too, often is related to excess weight. So also is high blood pressure.

In the very nature of risk factors, if you eliminate one, you cut your risk. But by eliminating one, you may at the same time be markedly influencing for the better a number of others.

How Much Does Inheritance Really Count? Is Coronary Heart Disease Inherited?

If one or both of your parents, your brothers or sisters, or one or both of your grandparents had heart attacks at early ages, the odds are greater that you will have a similar experience unless you do something to reduce them. But it's hardly a pure and simple matter of inheritance.

It can be very much a matter of environment—either acting on its own or interacting with inherited predispositions.

For example, is an obese person that way because he has inherited a tendency to be fat or because he comes from a family of big eaters? Eating habits are transmitted from parents to children and there is little reason to suspect that eating habits are genetically determined. It's a matter of exposure. A child of hearty-eating parents, if brought up in a family of moderate eaters, might well have no obesity problem at all. The obesity isn't in the genes.

We know that children of smoking parents are far more likely to smoke than the children of nonsmoking parents. There seems to be little evidence that there is some predisposition, genetically determined, to smoke. It is far more likely that smoking is an environmental matter.

Now let's go beyond that.

If a very high cholesterol level is found in your blood, it is likely that one or both of your parents—and quite likely some or all of your brothers and sisters, and your children as well—have high levels, too. Often the same is true for diabetes and high blood pressure.

So there may be hereditary predispositions for these problems. But the predispositions needn't invariably and inevitably lead to actualities. You may well not develop high cholesterol levels or diabetes or high blood pressure if certain environmental influences are changed so they differ from those acting on other members of your family. A change in diet could help, or a change in activity patterns, or other changes.

Even supposing that you have a very strong hereditary predisposition, strong enough to bring on a problem—high cholesterol, diabetes, or hypertension—without regard to environmental influences, you're still not licked. Such problems can be treated and overcome, or at least minimized as risk factors.

Moreover, there are the risk factors that are totally environmental in nature—smoking and sedentary living, for example—which you can control.

Are Birth Control Pills a Risk Factor?

Only for some women. Many millions of women use them with satisfaction and without serious side effects. But they do present a risk for some women who use them.

Research indicates that the risk is related to other known risk factors of heart disease. There may be particular risk for you if you smoke, have high blood pressure or a tendency toward it, a family history of heart attacks at an early age, a high level of blood lipids, a history of blood clots in the veins (phlebitis) or elsewhere, or, of course, heart disease itself.

If you have one or more of these risk factors, you should seriously consider—and discuss with your physician—whether the potential danger from oral contraceptives is worth the convenience, particularly if you are nearing the forties in age. There are, of course, other effective means of birth control that do not carry the risk.

If you should be using the Pill now and experience any chest distress, stop taking it immediately and see your physician—or go to a hospital emergency room without delay. Medicating yourself with painkillers or antacids could cost you your life.

What's the Evidence That Risk Factors Really Are Important?

Many studies—in the United States, Britain, and elsewhere—have made it clear that people with one or more of the factors have increased risk.

One of the most important studies that substantiated the importance of risk factors is known as the Framingham Study. Long-term and government-supported, the Framingham Study began in 1949 and still continues. It has been covering more than five thousand men and women in that Massachusetts community. All were healthy to begin with, and investigators have been keeping records of their health, of the illnesses they experienced, and of the development of angina and heart attacks. In addition, records have been kept of such matters as smoking, cholesterol and blood pressure levels, weight, eating habits, and living patterns.

The idea has been to see how the latter factors might or might not influence the development of disease.

The results of this study—the picture of the correlations between various factors and the development of coronary heart disease—can leave no doubt about the importance of these factors. For example, the Framingham Study (and studies elsewhere as well) has shown that men with blood cholesterol levels of 260 or higher have double the rate of new heart disease compared with the general population, while those with readings below 200 have only half the general rate. The study also found that smokers of two packs of cigarettes a day have an incidence of sudden death from heart attacks five times greater than that of nonsmokers. In addition, it was found that heavy smokers who give up smoking have after several years about the same incidence of heart attacks as men who have never smoked.

Similarly, in the Framingham research and in other studies, the increased risks for obesity, high blood pressure, and the other factors have been established.

HYPERTENSION: HIGH BLOOD PRESSURE AS A RISK FACTOR

If I Have Hypertension Will I Know It?

Not necessarily, because there may be no symptoms at all. The disease is subtle. Even when it does produce symptoms—such as headache, dizziness, fatigue, or weakness—these symptoms are common to many other problems. Hence, most cases of hypertension—or high blood pressure, which of course is what hypertension means—are not recognized by people who have it until it's discovered during the course of a physical examination.

For example, when employees at a large Michigan industrial plant were checked for hypertension, a large number were found to have it, although 78 percent of them had no idea they were hypertensive.

You can pretty much count on the fact that if you have elevated blood pressure the chances are you won't know you have it unless you're told so by a physician who checks it.

What, in Fact, Is Blood Pressure? When Is It Considered High?

Blood pressure is simply a force against the walls of your arteries. Each time your heart beats and pumps blood into the arteries to be distributed to the body, the pressure increases; in the interval between beats, the pressure goes down.

When your blood pressure is checked, the physican makes two readings and writes them in the form of a fraction—for example: 130/80. The first and larger figure is the systolic pressure, the pressure when the heart pumps; the second is the diastolic pressure, when the heart rests.

It's normal for blood pressure to fluctuate somewhat, decreasing when you rest or sleep, increasing when you're physically active or emotionally excited. And there is a considerable range of what is considered normal pressure. At rest, a systolic pressure in the 100-to-140 range and a diastolic in the 60-to-90 range is considered normal.

A single reading above 140/90 does not necessarily mean abnormal pressure. But when there is continuous elevation a person is considered to have hypertension.

Hypertension is common. By the lowest estimate, it affects 20 million Americans. Moreover, elevated pressure affects no one group of people in particular. It isn't a matter of age. Children, young adults, and middle-aged people, as well as the elderly, are affected.

Why Is Hypertension Dangerous?

For one thing, excessive pressure is a direct burden on the heart, which has to pump harder against the pressure. To meet the task, the heart may enlarge. Eventually the enlarged heart may weaken and become unable to circulate blood properly. This may cause the lungs to fill up with fluid and cause breathing difficulties, sleep problems, coughing spells during the night, or asthmatic wheezing.

Hypertension can also contribute to and accelerate atherosclerosis—the laying down of fatty deposits in the arteries feeding the heart.

Just as excessive water pressure in a garden hose may damage the hose after a time, so excessive pressure in the coronary arteries may damage the internal walls of the arteries, providing nesting places for any excess fats in the blood. Some investigators think that high pressure may even help force the fats into the walls to start the buildup of artery-narrowing deposits.

The effects of hypertension are not limited to the coronary arteries. Hypertension contributes greatly to stroke by accelerating atherosclerosis in brain arteries and to kidney disease by affecting the kidney arteries. In the Framingham Study, the risk of stroke has been found to be five times as high among people with even moderately elevated pressure levels (160/95) as among people with normal pressure.

To go back to coronary disease, not only does hypertension increase the risk that it will develop—tripling its incidence among men forty to fifty-five years of age, for example—but it also increases the deadliness of a heart attack when it comes. And in terms of coronary heart disease—and stroke, too—women do not tolerate hypertension any better than men.

What Causes Hypertension?

In 90 to 95 percent of cases, there is no detectable cause. In the remaining 5 to 10 percent the cause can be determined and a cure may be effected.

Where the cause is known, it may be a narrowing of a short segment of the aorta, the body's main trunk-line artery. Or there may be a tumor, commonly benign, of an adrenal gland atop a kidney. Or an abnormality in a kidney blood vessel, an accidental injury of a kidney, or an obstruction in a urinary duct. Inflammation or infection of the kidneys and the use of birth control pills may also cause hypertension.

When a cause can be found, medical or surgical treatment may cure the hypertension. For example, an adrenal gland tumor can be surgically removed and a diseased aorta or kidney vessel can also be surgically treated. When there is some likelihood that any such cause may exist, various tests—blood, urine,

X-ray studies of the kidney, chest, and some arteries—can be used to find it.

The vast majority of cases of high blood pressure, however, present no apparent cause—and these cases are known as *essential hypertension.* For essential hypertension, although there is no cure, effective control is almost always possible. Sometimes, diet may be enough for control; sometimes, medication is needed.

How Can Diet Help?

If you are overweight, the best treatment is weight reduction. There is a clear association between excess weight and hypertension. And for some people, getting rid of the excess is the only step necessary.

If you're hypertensive and overweight, you should be encouraged to lose the excess weight because, as we'll see, in addition to its asssociation with elevated blood pressure, which alone would make it important enough, excess weight can contribute in other ways to the increased risk of a fatal heart attack.

Admittedly, losing weight—and keeping it lost—is not a simple matter, especially in an age of crash and fad diets. Should a loss in weight fail to lower your pressure as much as necessary, your physician may prescribe medication.

What Kinds of Medication?

As a first step—and it may be the only step needed—you may receive a diuretic, or "water pill." Such a drug often helps. As it promotes the removal of excess fluid from body tissues, blood pressure tends to fall toward normal.

If a diuretic alone is not adequate, other medications may be added, drugs that act in various ways to lower blood pressure, in some cases by dampening down excessive nerve impulses that raise pressure, in other cases by helping to relax blood vessels.

Sometimes it's a simple matter to find the right drug or combination of drugs for a patient. Sometimes, it is more difficult, taking some trial and error to find a treatment regimen that accomplishes the desired pressure reduction with a minimum or absence of undesirable side effects.

Can Drug Side Effects Be Avoided?

To a large extent, yes.

There are many possible side effects—and different side effects with different people. Just as with foods, pollens, aspirin, and many other drugs, anti-hypertensive agents produce varying reactions depending on the individual. An anti-hypertensive drug may produce one side effect or several in one person, though none at all in another.

The side effects also vary from drug to drug. They range from sensations of lethargy, nasal stuffiness, dry mouth, and slight diarrhea to palpitations and effects on sexual function. More information about the side effects of anti-hypertensives will be found in Chapter 7, but I want to emphasize here that when bothersome side effects do occur, they may be transitory and may disappear as treatment continues. Sometimes a change in dosage may be effective, or a switch to another drug may be required.

There are now enough effective anti-hypertensives that your physician can arrive at a regimen that will help you without causing significant inconvenience.

Can Anything Be Done to Prevent Side Effects?

Yes. When you are taking drugs for hypertension, it's a good idea to avoid rapid changes in position—for example, when getting out of bed, getting up from a chair, or bending from the waist.

These motions, if sudden, may sometimes cause dizziness by producing a sudden temporary drop in blood pressure. Rather than jumping out of bed, sit briefly at the edge before standing up. If you have to pick up something from the floor, bend your knees; don't bend all the way from the waist.

Decreasing the Risks of Occurrence and Recurrence 91

It's also a good idea to avoid activities that may produce a sudden rise in blood pressure. These include undue excitement, of course, but also pushup exercises, weight lifting or other isometric-type exercises in which you briefly pit one muscle against another or against an immovable object.

If you are using a diuretic, it is possible that it will eliminate large amounts of potassium from the body. This may make you very tired. And if you should happen to need another drug, digitalis, for your heart, the loss of potassium may make you sensitive to otherwise useful levels of the digitalis, causing such symptoms as nausea, appetite loss, weakness, diarrhea, or slow or irregular heart rhythm.

So if you are using a diuretic, it's important that the level of potassium in your blood be checked by a simple test at regular intervals. And your physician may advise you to drink unsweetened orange juice regularly and perhaps eat a banana a day, since these fruits are rich in potassium. If food alone does not prevent a low level of potassium, potassium chloride medication may be needed.

Will I Need Medication for the Rest of My Life?

If medication is required to control your blood pressure, the chances are you will need to take it indefinitely.

What About Salt? Should It Be Eliminated from My Diet?

No, complete elimination of salt is usually not essential.

At one point, not too many years ago, there was little that could be done to help many hypertensives beyond rigid limitation of salt intake.

Studies have shown that high salt intake is related to hypertension. As early as 1948 a rice-and-fruit diet was being used with some good results to treat hypertension. What was the ingredient in the diet that accounted for the pressure-lowering? It turned out that the diet had no special ingredient but rather that it was very low in salt. And subsequently many studies showed that low salt intake could produce a lowering of blood pressure.

Almost complete removal of salt is not easy to accomplish or to live with. The average salt intake in the United States is about 15 grams, or half an ounce, a day. Severe salt restriction means limited intake to about 1/5 gram.

Diuretic drugs, not available in the 1940s, now control salt, eliminating excesses from the body. Nevertheless, moderation in use of salt may be desirable. Your physician may suggest limiting your salt intake to something on the order of 2 to 5 grams a day. That allows use of modest amounts of salt for cooking purposes but not the salting of foods at the table, but it requires avoidance of very salty foods such as crackers, potato chips, pretzels, processed meat, and ready-made sauces or seasoning extracts.

Can Biofeedback Help Reduce Blood Pressure?

Investigators at many institutions are checking on the possible value of biofeedback techniques. In biofeedback, electronic monitoring devices pick up internal signals and reveal to a patient—on a screen similar to a TV screen, or by audible signals—his or her blood pressure responses. Over a period of time, he or she may learn how to voluntarily control the autonomic nervous system so as to regulate blood pressure—in effect, "willing" the blood pressure lower.

The results are promising. Although in many cases biofeedback may not be adequate to bring the pressure all the way to normal, it sometimes may help, thus reducing the need for medication. Much more study is required before the true value of biofeedback is known.

Other efforts to find ways to reduce blood pressure without the need for drugs are being made. Some investigators have reported success in lowering blood pressure by means of a form of transcendental meditation called "relaxation response" or by psychotherapy.

Does It Really Pay Off to Lower Blood Pressure?

The value of modern drug treatment for hypertension has been dramatically demonstrated. As very high blood pressure has been reduced, enlarged hearts have decreased in size, signs and symptoms of heart failure have improved or even disappeared, kidney deterioration has been slowed or arrested, and the threat of stroke has diminished.

It remained for two Veterans Administration studies in seventeen VA hospitals across the country to show dramatically the value of drug therapy in both mild and moderate hypertension.

The results, first among moderate hypertensives, with diastolic pressures ranging from 115 to 129, were striking. Over an extended period, there were no deaths and only one nonfatal stroke and one nonfatal heart attack among those receiving treatment, contrasted with four deaths and twenty-seven serious heart attacks and strokes among others not receiving it.

In the second VA study, covering patients with diastolic pressures of 90 to 114, there was an impressive demonstration of the value of treatment for mild hypertension. Compared with other patients with such pressures not receiving treatment, those on drug treatment showed a two-thirds reduction in risk of stroke. The beneficial effect of such treatment on heart attacks has yet to be determined.

CHOLESTEROL AND BLOOD FATS AS A RISK FACTOR

What's the Difference Between Cholesterol and Blood Fats?

Cholesterol is one of the fatty materials, called lipids, found in the blood. It's virtually a household word by now.

Along with cholesterol, other lipids occur in the blood. They're known as triglycerides.

How Are Lipids Involved in Coronary Heart Disease?

Many studies have shown an association between the levels of the lipids and the occurrence of the disease.

It appears that virtually throughout the world, wherever groups of people have been investigated, those with relatively low occurrence rates of atherosclerosis and heart disease have been found to have relatively low levels of blood lipids.

Many investigations in the United States indicate that the risk of coronary heart disease rises sharply with increasing blood lipid levels.

The levels of lipids in the blood can be measured by simple tests and expressed in numbers. The Framingham Study, for example, has found that the frequency of coronary heart disease is seven times greater in persons with cholesterol values above 259 than among those with values below 200.

The Framingham Study, as well as other studies, also has pointed to the importance of triglyceride levels. The risk associated with high cholesterol level was found to increase if the triglyceride level was elevated. Even if the cholesterol level was moderate or low, the risk increased as the triglyceride level increased, and the opposite was equally true. Furthermore, people with high levels of both cholesterol and triglycerides seemed to be worse off than those with high levels of one or the other.

Do High Lipid Levels Always Mean Increased Risk?

There are some indications from recent studies—and these undoubtedly will now be investigated intensively—that another factor may enter the picture. That factor appears to be how cholesterol is transported in the body.

Cholesterol is carried about by chemicals called lipoproteins. One group of lipoproteins—called low-density lipoproteins, or LDLs—transports cholesterol from the liver to the cells of the body where it is used to help make cell membranes and certain hormones. A second group of lipoproteins—called high-density lipoproteins, or HDLs—clears away unneeded cholesterol from body tissues and returns it to the liver for excretion from the body.

The available evidence suggests that when high blood cholesterol levels are linked to high levels of LDLs, there is increased risk of clogging of arteries and heart disease. On the other hand, it appears that if the high cholesterol levels are linked to high HDL levels, there may be less risk of artery and heart disease; there is even some possibility that high HDL levels may protect against disease.

Especially as more information is obtained about the significance of the lipoprotein factor, it may be taken into consideration. If you have a high cholesterol level, your physician may order further tests to determine whether the seemingly protective HDLs or the dangerous LDLs are responsible for those elevated levels. A simple test is now commercially available. By subtracting the HDLs from the total cholesterol, the LDLs can be estimated. A ratio of HDLs and LDLs favoring the HDLs seems to be favorable for avoiding atherosclerosis. Exercise, loss of weight, and low-cholesterol diet influence the ratio favorably; smoking and inactivity, unfavorably.

How Is Lipid Level Tested?

It's a very simple procedure for the patient, involving taking a small sample of blood from a vein. The test should be done after fasting for at least fourteen hours, so it can be done in the morning prior to breakfast after an overnight fast. It's also best done after you have been on your regular diet, whatever it may be, for several weeks prior to the test. It should not be done shortly after a heart attack.

Do Lipids Serve Useful Purposes?

They certainly do.

Fats are stored in the body mainly in the form of triglycerides. They are stored, among other reasons, because they hold a lot of concentrated energy. When the body needs energy, the fats can be mustered and carried as triglycerides in the blood to where the energy is needed.

Cholesterol, too, is a vital material. It is contained in almost every cell of the body and it may have a role in regulating the passage of nutrient materials into and out of the cell through the cell membranes.

There is a high concentration of cholesterol in the brain, and it may act there in some important though not yet understood capacity.

Moreover, cholesterol serves as a material from which other important body materials are manufactured. For example, the corticosteroids (hormones of the adrenal gland such as cortisone) are produced from cholesterol. So are the sex hormones. Cholesterol is also changed by the body to bile acids and excreted in the bile that flows into the intestine to help in the digestion of fats.

So certain levels of both cholesterol and triglycerides in the blood, which transports them both, are normal and essential. It's when those levels become abnormally elevated that the risk of atherosclerosis and heart disease increases.

If the Cholesterol Level Is Elevated, Is the Triglyceride Level Elevated, Too?

Not necessarily. In many cases, both are elevated; in many others, one may be elevated while the other is at normal level. In fact, physicians classify hyperlipemia (elevated blood fats) into five groups and even some technical subdivisions.

In Type I hyperlipemia, which is relatively rare, cholesterol is only slightly elevated but triglyceride is greatly elevated.

Type II is more common. Here cholesterol is up but triglyceride is not.

In Type III, which like Type I is not very common, both cholesterol and triglyceride levels are up.

Type IV is common. Cholesterol may be normal but the triglyceride level is up.

In Type V, not as common as Types II and IV, sometimes cholesterol level is only a bit high, sometimes very high. But always the triglyceride level is way up.

What Can Be Done to Lower High Cholesterol Levels?

Diet can be valuable.

Dietary control is based upon two principles. The first principle is that foods vary greatly in their content of cholesterol and that cholesterol intake can be reduced by proper food selection.

The cholesterol content of foods is measured in milligrams of cholesterol in 100-gram (3½-ounce) portions. Among foods especially high in cholesterol are egg yolk (with 1,500 milligrams per 100 grams), butter (250), kidney (375), sweetbreads (250), calf brains (2,000 plus), and lobster (200).

On the other hand, some foods have very little or almost no cholesterol content at all. Among them are fruits, vegetables, egg whites, cereals, vegetable oils, peanut butter, and vegetable margarine. Skim milk and milk powder are very low in cholesterol.

What's the Second Principle of Dietary Control of High Cholesterol?

It's based on the finding that the lower the ratio between saturated and unsaturated fats in the diet, the lower the cholesterol level is likely to be. When the association between high blood cholesterol levels and artery disease was first noted, attempts were made to try to reduce the levels only by reducing cholesterol intake in the diet. But it turned out that the reduced intake wasn't enough to bring down the levels to any marked extent.

Next came the finding that the amount of fats in the diet does matter. Individuals who were placed on a low-cholesterol diet but a diet still high in fats continued to have elevated cholesterol levels. And after considerable research it was found that fat in the diet seemed to facilitate the absorption by the body of cholesterol in food.

Even so, when a low-fat diet was tried, it did not invariably lead to blood cholesterol reduction. It took further research to determine that it was the *type* of fat that counted.

There are three distinctive types of fats:

Saturated fats, which tend to increase blood cholesterol

levels, are fats that harden at room temperatures, such as gravy fat. Saturated fats occur in many meats, particularly beef, lamb, and pork. They occur, too, in butter, cream, whole milk, and cheeses made from cream and whole milk. And there are saturated vegetable fats; they occur in many solid and hydrogenated shortenings, and in the coconut oil, cocoa butter, and palm oil commonly used in commercially made cookies, pie fillings, and nondairy milk and cream substitutes.

Polyunsaturated fats, which tend to lower blood cholesterol levels, are fats that remain liquid at room temperature. Among them are such oils as corn, cottonseed, safflower, sesame seed, soybean, and sunflower seed.

Monounsaturated fats are a third type. They seem to have little if any effect on blood cholesterol levels. Olive oil is an example.

How Do I Apply the Principles to My Diet?

You can apply them with moderate rather than drastic changes in what may now be your dietary pattern.

Because egg yolks are very rich in cholesterol, your physician may suggest limiting your intake of egg yolks to perhaps one or two a week, including yolks used in prepared food. There need be no limits on use of egg whites in cooking; they are largely made up of protein.

Your physician may also suggest that in your choice of dairy products you emphasize such foods as skim milk, buttermilk, cottage cheese, and other cheeses low in fat (such as farmer and hoop), choosing these in place of other cheeses, butter, ice cream, and sweet and sour cream.

Lovers of steaks, chops, roasts, and shellfish don't have to give them up entirely but should eat smaller portions and have them as entrees less often. When you have such meat dishes, you can trim away visible fat and, in the case of roasts, discard dripping fat rather than using it for gravy. You can also eat less fried and more roasted, broiled, baked, and boiled meat.

As you cut down on steaks, chops, roasts, and shellfish you

Decreasing the Risks of Occurrence and Recurrence 99

can make greater use of chicken and turkey, avoiding the skin, where the fat is largely concentrated. And you can make more use of fish.

If you like soups, eat those that don't contain a lot of fat. You can often eliminate much of the fat by refrigerating a soup after cooking it, then skimming off the fat at the top before reheating.

Your physician may well suggest, too, that you eat more vegetables, salads, and fruits. They are generally low in calories and fats, high in vitamins and minerals, and helpful in moderating your appetite through their bulk.

You need not eliminate desserts entirely but you should eat smaller portions and eat them less often, perhaps using fruits as substitutes frequently.

Quite possibly, you may be referred to the American Heart Association's fat-controlled, low-cholesterol meal plan. If so, you will find it in Appendix D.

The plan has several objectives. It aims at avoiding excessive quantities of cholesterol and saturated fats by reducing your intake of foods that are especially rich in them and at having you eat more of the polyunsaturated fats, and less of the saturated. At the same time, it tries to fulfill your daily needs for proteins, vitamins, minerals, and other essential nutrients, and also to control calories and help you maintain a desirable weight.

The plan does all this while still providing a considerable variety of foods, very likely including many of your favorites.

Can Dietary Measures Control Elevated Triglyceride Levels?

Very often, yes.

In some cases, however, the elevation seems to be an inherited tendency. More often, abnormal triglyceride levels are associated with excess weight. Not uncommonly, in obese people, weight reduction alone brings down the levels.

Excessive use of sugar and alcohol may be involved, and reduction of their intake may be effective.

Our use of sugar overall—in the United States and in most Western nations—is fantastically high. Until about a century ago, very little sugar was used. It was a luxury, sold by the ounce—virtually on a par with caviar. Then came the development of methods of refining sugar from beets, and it stopped being a luxury. Today, sugar intake for the average American runs well above two pounds a week.

It isn't alone a matter of the sugar we add to coffee and tea and to cereals and fruits. Sugar is found in a great variety of prepared foods and beverages—in cakes, pies, pastries, candies, jams, jellies, ice cream, and gelatin desserts. Not uncommonly, soft drinks contain as much as 10 percent sugar. And sugar is often contained now in salad dressings, vegetable juices, soups, and some other canned foods.

The huge consumption of sugar has long been of concern—at first largely in connection with dental disease. That sugar plays a significant role in dental decay, feeding the bacteria that attack tooth enamel, has long been well established.

Sugar has been indicted, too, as an important influence in the obesity problem. It is, after all, an "empty calorie" food. It contains no proteins, vitamins, or minerals—only calories. With so many of us leading relatively sedentary, inactive lives, there seems to be little if any reason to have something in the diet that provides only calories that we don't need.

Not without good reason, it has been suggested that many people could avoid excess weight or get rid of it by restricting sugar. Say you take just one spoonful of sugar in each cup of coffee or tea and drink only five cups a day. Just by eliminating the sugar in your coffee or tea, you could lose several pounds in a year.

So your doctor may well suggest that you try to eliminate or reduce your sugar intake as a help in bringing down elevated triglyceride levels and in keeping your weight at a desirable level.

Is There Medication I Can Take to Lower My Blood Lipids If They Are Too High?

It was believed until recently that certain drugs could bring down elevated blood lipid levels and in so doing improve the outlook for heart patients. But the Coronary Drug Project, a nationwide study carried out at fifty-three medical centers, has cast some doubt on this.

Lipid-lowering drugs—such as estrogen, dextrothyroxine, nicotinic acid, and clofibrate—were used in patients who had experienced previous heart attacks. The comprehensive study found that the drugs were not helpful in preventing recurrent heart attacks and frequently had serious side effects.

The Coronary Drug Project results differ from those of two previous British studies which found that clofibrate may be effective in reducing repeat heart attacks and deaths.

We hope that medical research can produce drugs that can be effective in preventing or helping to prevent heart attacks by reducing blood lipid levels without producing any serious side effects.

Meanwhile, let me add that while general adherence to a low-fat, low-cholesterol, and low-sugar diet is advisable, you should not become unduly alarmed about a high lipid level, fearful that it must inevitably affect you adversely. Other risk factors are important and very often controllable.

OVERWEIGHT AS A RISK FACTOR

Is Excess Weight Really a Significant Risk Factor?

It is. In the Framingham Study, for example, among men who were 30 percent overweight, there was a 2.8 times greater risk of developing coronary heart disease within ten years than among those who were 10 percent or more underweight.

How may overweight help to promote coronary heart disease? For one thing, it adds to the heart's work load since circulation is provided for the fatty tissue. And it is also a fact that high blood pressure is often present in someone who is overweight and that blood lipid abnormalities tend to be more common, too.

In addition, in the total picture, excess weight has adverse effects on many other diseases.

Insurance data, collected over many years, indicates that excess mortality—from all causes—increases rapidly with increasing degree of overweight. For example, the excess death rate is 13 percent for men who are 10 percent overweight. The rate increases to 25 percent for those 20 percent overweight, and to 40 percent for those 30 percent overweight. For women, excess weight also increases mortality: there is a 30 percent excess mortality rate among women who are 30 percent overweight.

These are insurance figures for some specific diseases. As compared with the population in general, overweight men and women have these excesses of mortality: for heart attacks, 142 percent and 175 percent respectively; for stroke, 159 percent and 162 percent; for chronic nephritis (kidney disease), 191 percent and 212 percent; for diabetes, 383 percent and 372 percent.

What Should I Weigh If I'm to Reduce Risk?

You'll find a table of desirable weights for men and women in Appendix A. This will give you some guidance. It may be all you need, unless you happen to be exceptional.

It is possible for some people to be overweight without actually having any excess fat—as is the case, for example, with some college football players. And, on the other hand, some people, particularly the very sedentary, may be carrying excess fat even though they are not markedly overweight.

As a check, you can use a few simple tests. One is the ruler test. Usually, if there is no excess fat, you will have a flat abdominal surface between the point where your ribs flare out and the front of the pelvis. For the test, lie on your back and place a ruler on the abdomen along the midline of the body. If it points upward at the midsection, that can be an indication you may be carrying too much fat.

The pinch test may also be useful. With your thumb and forefinger you can grasp a "pinch" of skin—at the stomach, upper arm, buttocks, and calf. Much of body fat is located directly under the skin. Generally, that under-skin layer, which is what you measure with the pinch, should be between ¼ and ½ inch.

With the pinch, of course, you're measuring a double thickness—and that, normally, should be between ½ inch and 1 inch. A fold much more than 1 inch indicates excess fat.

Very likely, you'll have no difficulty deciding whether or not you are overweight. If you do, your doctor, of course, will be glad to provide further guidance.

But If I'm Overweight, It's Not Easy to Reduce—How Do I Do That Effectively?

It isn't easy, but it may be less difficult than you imagine. Your doctor will undoubtedly guide you—and warn you against fad diets, which can be worse than useless.

There's no question but that various highly publicized diets that gain popularity from time to time—some of them repeatedly under different names—can take weight off and even take it off quickly, though often much of the weight lost is water. However, the losses are temporary and useless, except perhaps for some brief cosmetic appeal. Weight-reducing drugs, too, have only short-term effects, are often dangerous, and are rarely indicated.

What's needed is not to take off much weight rapidly with some temporarily effective diet. Instead, you need to lose a little—half a pound or a pound a week—and do it with dietary modifications that, to a large extent, you can live with for the rest of your life.

There is no escaping the fact that except in very rare instances when there may be some physical problem such as a gland disorder, excess weight results from taking in more calories than are expended. Taking off weight requires taking in fewer calories than are expended—and, thereafter, keeping weight at a desirable level requires matching intake and expenditure.

One pound of body fat represents 3,500 calories. And to lose that pound you have to establish a 3,500 calorie deficit.

A sound reducing diet should lead to the loss of as many pounds as necessary at a safe rate over a reasonable period. It should, at the same time, provide balanced and varied eating so that your health is maintained and so that you get some pleasure in eating as well as some satisfaction of hunger.

And, not least of all, it should establish eating patterns that are enjoyable, tolerable, and conducive to being maintained. To be sure, after you have lost the desirable number of pounds, you can add a little to your intake. But the last thing you want to do is revert to old eating habits that produced the excess weight in the first place.

Usually, along with a sound diet for weight reduction and proper weight maintenance thereafter, a good program of physical activity can be valuable if your physician okays that for you. By increasing calorie expenditures, physical activity helps minimize the need for calorie restrictions. And it can do much more—contributing to general fitness and vigor, and, as we'll see, to cardiovascular health.

How Do I Go About Reducing?

By all means let your physican help and guide. He or she may suggest that you make use of some of the tools I'm including in this book.

As I noted earlier, there has to be a deficit of 3,500 calories to take off a pound of excess weight. Thus, a daily deficit of 500 calories can produce a weight loss of a pound in a week. Your physician may suggest that this is the correct pace for you, or may advise a lesser or greater daily deficit to fit your needs.

Your physician may well determine, too, to what extent the deficit is to be achieved by reduced calorie intake and to what extent by increased calorie expenditure. If yours has been a quite sedentary life-style, he or she may urge more physical activity and tailor a program for you—as a help for more than weight reduction alone.

Let's say that, for example, you are advised to add half an hour of walking a day. That would mean expending about 150 more calories a day than you have been doing. If the prescribed deficit to be achieved is 500 calories a day, that leaves 350 calories to be cut out of daily food intake.

Your physician then can help you to determine what your total caloric intake should be. There's a simple general rule to use for this. Generally, it takes about 15 calories a day to maintain a pound of body weight for a person doing average work. That being the case, if you weigh, say, 150 pounds, you need 2,250 calories a day to maintain present weight. And if you want to reduce at the rate of a pound a week and therefore with a calorie deficit of 500 a day, with 150 calories taken care of by activity, leaving 350 calories to come out of food intake, you need a daily diet that will provide 1,900 calories.

So it will be helpful for you to become familiar with the caloric values of various foods, and you will find these in the table in Appendix B.

But you have to consider more than calories alone in setting up a proper diet. The diet should be balanced and varied, containing suitable amounts of proteins, carbohydrates, and fats. Such a diet can provide suitable quantities of vitamins, minerals, and other essential nutrients.

And it should help in controlling blood lipids. Your physician may suggest, then, that you use the American Heart Association fat-controlled, low-cholesterol meal plan in Appendix D in conjunction with the calorie table as a guide. And, of course, he can help you in setting up your dietary regimen.

Your doctor may also, if he believes it will be helpful for you, prescribe an American Heart Association booklet that is available only on prescription: *Planning Fat-Controlled Meals for 1200 and 1800 Calories.* It uses the same principles as those in the plan in Appendix D and includes sample menus and useful recipes for both 1,200- and 1,800-calorie diets.

Perhaps you've dieted repeatedly in the past. This time, let it be effective dieting in which you aim for and achieve long-term results.

SEDENTARY LIVING AS A RISK FACTOR

If I Lead a Sedentary Life, Am I More Likely to Have a Heart Problem Than If I Lead an Active Life?

Many studies suggest that sedentary living—lack of physical activity—may be a risk factor. It appears that physical activity is of value, even though it is certainly not the whole answer, in helping to protect against heart problems.

For example, in England, bus conductors who climb up and down double-decker buses have been found to have less heart disease than drivers of the same buses.

Also in England, and in Scotland and Wales, a national autopsy survey produced additional evidence to support the theory that men in physically active work have less coronary heart disease than those in more sedentary occupations. Five thousand autopsy reports were studied and the job activities of each subject were considered. It turned out that not only did physically active men—postmen, laborers, and others—have less coronary heart disease than such sedentary workers as schoolteachers but also that the disease they had was less severe and developed later.

Similar studies have been done in the United States. For example, one investigation of 120,000 railroad employees found the incidence of heart attacks almost twice as great among the office workers as among the men working in the yards. A study of District of Columbia postal workers showed that clerks had 1.4 times the risk of coronary heart disease as the mail carriers.

Could a Program of Exercise Help Me?

If it's a good program—and we'll discuss that soon—very probably it will help. Almost certainly it will help you to feel better, to feel fit and more healthy generally.

A good program of exercise may decrease angina and increase your work capacity. If you are in good physical condition, your heart rate and blood pressure will rise less with a given amount of physical work than if you are not. Physical activity also tends to increase the high-density lipoproteins that recent studies suggest may be valuable in decreasing atherosclerosis. Some scientists even believe that properly planned exercise may prolong life, although this point is not yet proven.

An exercise program may make a contribution to your heart and blood vessel health by helping to combat other risk factors.

How May It Contribute to Combating Other Risk Factors?

We've already discussed the problem of overweight and noted that exercise can help in solving it. But the subject is important enough—and so often misunderstood—that I think it is worthwhile to spend just a little more time on it.

Exercise is as much linked to weight as food is. It's difficult for many of us to appreciate how sedentary our contemporary living is, how relatively little energy we expend unless we deliberately seek ways to expend it.

Even farmers today ride tractors where once they walked. The housewife today no longer scrubs floors or washes clothes at an energy expenditure on the order of 250 calories an hour; instead, she uses washing machines, vacuum cleaners, and other modern devices at an output of perhaps 120 calories an hour.

Not long ago, one British physiologist observed: "Even young military cadets spend 17¾ hours a day either lying, sitting, or standing; the corresponding figure for coal miners is 18¾ hours a day.... Military cadets and miners have two of the most physically active occupations, and yet about three quarters of their life is sedentary."

Very probably you have heard an old myth repeated many times—that exercise is a negligible factor in avoiding or overcoming obesity. To no small extent it may result from misunderstandings of some often-cited statistics—such as that it takes five hours of wood chopping, and even more walking, to lose a pound.

Now that, of course, would make exercise as a weight-reducer seem simply impractical. Nobody has the time for all the exercise that would be needed, and the implication is that it would be insane to even consider it.

But put it in context.

Yes, you have to burn up 3,500 calories to lose a pound. But you don't have to do the burning all at once. You don't put on excess weight that way—all at once. You can gain something on the order of eight pounds in one year simply by eating one extra pat of butter a day. Or you can add just one piece of pie per week and can gain three pounds or more in a year.

In the same way, when it comes to using exercise to control weight, a little increase in activity each day can accomplish a lot in a year. With an increased expenditure of 200 calories a day, the expenditure in a year would equal 73,000 calories, enough to eliminate twenty excess pounds.

A daily walk of less than an hour can use up 200 calories for most people. The actual expenditure, of course, depends upon the speed and the weight of the individual. A 150-pound person, for example, walking at three miles an hour will consume 120 calories in half an hour. If he or she is heavier or walks faster or both, the expenditure goes higher.

Does Exercise Have Any Effect on Blood Lipids?

There are indications in animal and human studies that exercise does have a beneficial effect. Rabbits, for example, have been divided into two groups, both receiving diets rich in cholesterol. One group was vigorously exercised; the other, not. Upon examination, the exercised animals had lower cholesterol levels.

A Harvard diet-exercise study involved three medical students. To begin with, the students' caloric intake was doubled while they exercised vigorously. As long as they continued the exercise, they gained no weight and had no increase in blood fat levels. But when the exercising was stopped and the same high caloric intake continued, both weight and blood fat levels increased.

At Kent State University, a researcher worked with forty-two men ranging in age from twenty-nine to sixty-three, all in sedentary occupations. For an hour a day, five days a week, for nine months, they took part in an intensive physical fitness program. In every man, blood cholesterol declined, with the biggest decline occurring in those with the highest levels at the beginning.

More recently, in Palo Alto, California, where Stanford University has a Heart Disease Prevention Program, investigators studied forty-one men, aged thirty-five to fifty-nine, who averaged fifteen miles of running a week. Many had begun to run only in the last few years. Blood fat levels in these men were more like those of young women least vulnerable to heart disease than those of sedentary middle-aged men. Blood cholesterol levels were significantly lower and blood triglyceride levels were only half those of men of comparable age leading sedentary lives.

Is Hypertension Affected by Exercise?

There are studies which suggest that physical activity can help to lower elevated blood pressure at least a little.

In one study, for example, researchers at the San Diego State College Exercise Laboratory placed twenty-three hypertensive men on a moderate exercise program. It consisted of 15 to 20 minutes of warm-up calisthenics and no more than 30 to 35 minutes of walking-jogging twice a week. Before the program, the average blood pressure for the group was 159/105. After six months on the program, it was 148/93.

Does Exercise Have Any Effect on Tension?

Tension and stress are considered to be risk factors, and physical activity may serve to ease them.

You may have noticed, in your own experience, that if you're wound up over a problem, anxious about it, perhaps frustrated at least for the moment, you may feel almost a violent need to get up and move about, *not* to sit still. And perhaps you've noted that it's difficult, if not impossible, to stay wound up with some worry or concern when you're playing a game of tennis or jogging or bowling or batting a ball with the kids.

It's common experience, everyday observation, that physical activity does seem to be relaxing. A physiological reason for this has been suggested, based on the concept of stress: when you become tense and anxious, the adrenal glands atop the kidneys respond by pouring out hormone secretions that are designed to ready you to fight or flee. You're mobilized, in effect, for physical action.

You might say that this is a carryover from the time when our ancient ancestors became tense and anxious, usually in situations of physical emergency—when, for example, they were confronted with a dangerous animal or a storm or other natural danger. To live, they had to react quickly, either by standing up to the danger or running from it. The increased adrenal gland secretions provided the extra energy for this.

Today, of course, we rarely face the same kind of emergencies. Far more often, when we become tense and anxious, it's because of some problem or pressure we can't respond to by fighting or fleeing. Instead, we're likely to sit and become wound up.

You could say that we are indeed wound up with a lot of energy churning around inside that we don't, and even can't, direct outward as our ancestors did, at least not in terms of the tension-causing situation.

But it may be possible to work off some or much of that energy—and tension—by physical activity.

What Can Exercise Do for the Heart Itself?

It may have more than one beneficial effect.

As you know, the heart is a muscle, and, as for any other muscle, exercise can help to make the heart more efficient.

If you exercise, say, the muscles of your arms, they will grow in time, become stronger and more efficient. The same is true for the heart. A trained athlete's heart is enlarged because the heart muscle fibers gradually enlarge. Because the fibers enlarge, the ventricles—or pumping chambers of the heart—enlarge. They can hold and pump more blood.

As a result, when an athlete is resting, his heart, with its increased capacity, doesn't have to pump as often. Commonly, the heart rate of a trained athlete at rest is much lower than, sometimes only half, that of a more sedentary person.

During vigorous activity, an athlete's heart responds readily, contracting more completely with each beat to pump out more blood. The heart rate doesn't have to increase as much as in a sedentary person—and once the activity is over the heart rate slows down again far more rapidly than the heart rate of an unfit individual.

Heart specialists a few years ago became intrigued by the Tarahumara Indians of Mexico. The tribe has a favorite game of kick-ball. Trained from childhood, men and women participants in the game can run continuously for over 100 miles at a speed of six to seven miles an hour while pursuing and kicking a wooden ball.

Physicians intensively studied eight of the runners, men aged eighteen to forty-eight. Their blood pressures were checked in the middle of a long kick-ball race and were found to have decreased markedly from what they were at the start. At the same time, pulse rates had risen to a range of 120 to 155. The average weight loss during the race was five pounds. Extensive tests after the race showed no abnormal changes of any kind. None of the tribe could recall a single instance in which a runner had dropped out of a race because of chest pain or shortness of breath.

One of the physician-investigators, a professor of medicine and associate dean of the University of Oklahoma Medical Center, has remarked: "These marathon demonstrations of really phenomenal endurance are convincing evidence that most of us, brought up in our comfortable and sedentary civilizations, actually develop and use only a fraction of our potential cardiac reserve."

Does Exercise Have Other Possible Value for the Heart?

You'll recall that in Chapter 3, page 50, we noted that in a heart attack the very minute a coronary artery feeding the heart is choked off, the body is stimulated to develop small new blood vessels—collaterals—to help bring blood to the area around the damaged muscle and, in so doing, to help in the healing process.

The collateral circulation development during a heart attack results, in effect, from the sudden stress brought on by the attack.

It's believed by many investigators that exercise over an extended period of time provides a kind of controlled stress that may also lead to the development of collateral vessels. This, of course, would be very desirable.

It's even possible that, if collateral circulation is great enough, a heart attack may be prevented, since a spare vessel might be able to take over immediately when a coronary artery or branch becomes blocked, with virtually no blood flow interruption, and therefore little if any damage to the heart muscle.

It has been suggested, too, that collateral circulation may be the reason that some people do not suffer from anginal chest pain even though they have severe atherosclerosis. It would seem that even though blood flow through the diseased arteries has been diminished increasingly, it has been counterbalanced by flow through the collaterals.

In the Framingham Study, greater mortality from coronary heart disease was observed among the sedentary, who also were especially prone to sudden death. The findings suggested that the greater protection enjoyed by the physically active could result at least to some extent from the development of collateral circulation.

Are There Still Other Possible Values of Exercise?

Some are, of course, well known. Exercise can increase general muscular strength and endurance, and may in time help to overcome easy fatigue or feelings of listlessness. Exercise has also been used to correct postural defects.

The results of an unusual study carried out in the sleep laboratory of the State University of New York Downstate Medical Center, Brooklyn, are interesting. Investigators checked on the sleep of fourteen normal college students used to regular exercise.

Their sleep was monitored with instruments on two nights after they had had their usual exercise and then on four nights during a one-month period when all exercise was prohibited.

The subjects complained that they didn't sleep as well during the month without exercise. And on the four nights when their sleep was monitored, the recordings showed changes in the sleep pattern indicative of increased anxiety. It was also reported that during the month without exercise the students experienced increased sexual tension.

Don't People Reach an Age at Which They're Too Old for Exercise?

That is a serious misconception. In fact, many false assumptions have been made about aging and physical vigor.

Among them have been assumptions that aging must inevitably bring physical decline; that such decline can neither be prevented nor remedied; that with age one becomes inherently incapable of exertion and that exercise and activity not only are largely beyond the capacities of the elderly but even dangerous, harmful rather than beneficial.

All of these are belied by the many older people who are vigorously active. You can see them out jogging, running, bicycling, swimming, playing tennis, and engaging in other physical activities and sports. They may not have the same stamina as eighteen-year-olds, but they have more than many of the overfed, underexercised young adults.

Many studies, including some being conducted at the University of Southern California's Gerontology Center, indicate that people in their sixties and seventies and even beyond can retain, with carefully planned exercise, much of the vigor of their forties. It has also been shown that well-planned exercise programs can be rehabilitative, sometimes strikingly so.

Several years ago, Senator Jennings Randolph reported, in the Congressional Record, on a demonstration he had witnessed in Charleston, West Virginia, while conducting a hearing for the Senate Committee on Aging. He had watched a group of older people—ages sixty-five to eighty-five—go through vigorous calisthenics. All were suffering from chronic conditions or recovering from acute physical disabilities that had made them almost completely immobile. That, however, was before they began participating in a program of Physical Fitness for Senior Citizens developed by the Lawrence Frankel Foundation of Charleston and carried out under medical supervision.

Only six months after beginning a series of supervised and individualized calisthenics classes, they had become able to participate in community activities and have social contacts instead of watching from the sidelines in loneliness and depression, as Randolph noted. The program was a pilot project on which a statewide plan for physical fitness programs for the elderly might be based.

A sixty-nine-year-old woman, who had been sick with heart disease a year before, had suffered from spinal arthritis and a nerve ailment, and had required sleeping pills nightly, put on a demonstration of sit-ups, strength exercises and balancing on a balance beam. She hasn't needed a sleeping pill since starting the program.

Interestingly, there is a theory that proposes that older people may have a special need for exercise, that physical activity may have profound psychological value for them.

Why Is There a Special Need Among Older People?

A study by two Israeli psychologists developed the theory that all of us start out, as children, relishing movement. Almost universally, children enjoy movement just for the sake of moving. When they discover some new pattern of motion, they get pleasure out of performing it—in play, sports, dancing, and other activities—to the point of satiation.

But for sedentary elderly people, pleasure from movement is steadily reduced. Eventually, they may become reluctant to move at all. And beyond leading to muscular degeneration, such inactivity may lead to psychological changes.

An important psychological change suggested by the study

is distortion of body image. Physically inactive people over fifty, the study indicates, perceive their bodies to be heavier and broader than they really are. And, exactly because of this distorted perception, they come to look upon bodily movements as increasingly strenuous.

They may then be caught in a vicious cycle. Looking upon movements as more and more strenuous, they make less and less effort to move, and that only adds further to the distortion of body image, which then leads to greater clumsiness and fear of activity.

Moreover, the study suggests, with no physical outlet for discharging energy, internal tension in the elderly increases. And this increase is piled on top of internal tension caused by pent-up aggression.

Certainly, aggressive tendencies are not confined to the elderly. Younger people have them, together with more opportunities to release their energies, to direct their aggressive tendencies outward, through bodily movements.

But older people have more difficulty expressing aggression, for one thing, because they may be more introverted. Moreover, society, with its stereotypes for "proper" behavior in the elderly, tends to immobilize them. Older people are not expected to dance rock and roll or even to ride a bicycle. Rather, the older person is expected to be "dignified," which seems to be synonymous with confining oneself to restrained movement.

The buildup of tension in the elderly, the study suggests, can produce such symptoms as insomnia, fretfulness, and restlessness. Thus, the elderly often may turn their unreleased aggressive tendencies inward upon themselves—and these may become self-destructive, leading to depression which, in turn, may increase tendencies toward psychosomatic diseases or lead to sudden outbursts of rage.

Regular bodily exercise, according to the research, can provide emotional satisfaction: it can break the vicious cycle in which body image distortions caused by inactivity lead to more inactivity and further distortions; it can use up energies that need to be used up and prevent internalization of aggression.

As I have indicated, this is a theory—and must remain a theory until definite proof is established. But it is rational, and provocative.

But Can't Exercise Be Dangerous?

Of course it can be—for young and for old—unless it is approached sensibly.

An all-out, sudden burst of activity after many years—even just many months—of relative inactivity can cause great aches and pains. It can also be lethal, placing sudden great strain on the heart. Exercises that unduly elevate blood pressure and heart rate may be particularly dangerous and should be avoided by high-risk patients. Such exercises include push-ups, weight lifting, shoveling snow, vacuum cleaning, cutting grass, raking leaves, expanding or compressing springs, moving heavy objects, and trying to open stuck doors or windows.

What Would Be a Sensible Approach for Me?

By all means, consult your physician first. Let him or her check you and advise you as to whether you are able at this point to undertake a program of exercise.

That's advisable for even a young adult who has long led a sedentary life. It's certainly even more so if you have had a heart attack or suffer from angina or have other indications of coronary heart disease. If you have been ill or if you have a heart condition, generally the best way to get started is by walking.

Walking is underrated. It involves many muscles. It is a continuous type of activity. And it is valuable, too, because it lends itself to a slow start and a progressive, unstraining buildup of effort.

There are also certain key principles your physician probably will urge you to follow.

What Precautionary Rules Do You Advise?

The first is tolerance, which means that you should make no sudden great demand on your body, that you should avoid excessive straining.

The second is overload. That means that after you have become accustomed to a level of activity, have developed tolerance for it, then you go just a little further, exercise just a little harder. This applies to walking, jogging, swimming, bicycling, or any form of exercise. Let's amplify that a bit. At first, you walk or jog or whatever at a comfortable pace only until you first begin to feel tired. Then you go a little beyond—exercising a little longer or harder—beyond the first feeling of being tired. Only a little—until you gradually develop a tolerance for that level of activity.

The next important principle is progression. As you become regularly active, your strength and endurance will gradually increase. Your activities then become easier for you. If you continue to carry them out at the same pace or for the same time period, you will be maintaining your improvement. To increase it, you can, with your physician's advice, build up further on your activities, making them progressively more strenuous, always a little at a time.

What's the Best Program?

There isn't any one that is best.

It is important that your program be a balanced and, at least at the beginning, a supervised one. It should be devoted not only to building up one or a few muscles—abdominal muscles, biceps, or whatever—but also to providing some training for the heart and circulation. For this, the best activities are those that are continuous and involve larger muscle groups—such as brisk walking, swimming, and jogging. Swimming should be near the edge of the water, not after meals, not in too cold water, and with gradual entrance into the water.

If you include a continuous activity along with any exercises for special muscles that you may be interested in, you will have a balanced program.

When it comes to a continuous activity, your physician may suggest, for example, that you start with a few minutes of walking daily, beginning at a relatively leisurely pace ("warming up") and progressively making it brisker. He may then suggest that you add, gradually, a few more minutes of walking daily. After brisk walking—or any vigorous physical effort—sudden cessation of activity may be harmful and must be avoided by a gradual decrease of such activity ("cooling off"). If exercise causes angina, it should be interrupted. Patients with angina are better off taking nitroglycerin as a preventive measure before exercise. Later, after they become conditioned, they may no longer need it.

After a time you may feel like occasionally breaking up your walking with a brief period of jogging. Some physicians may suggest that you gradually jog more and more and walk less and less until finally you may be spending all your continuous activity period in jogging. Jogging, however, at least at the beginning, should be done only under strict supervision, with all emergency treatment readily available. The local heart association usually is able to guide you to such a physical activity program.

All exercise, at least initially, must be supervised by monitoring the increase of heart rate and any possible disturbance of heart rhythm. If a particular exercise leads to undue heart rate increase or a significant rhythm disturbance, it is best discontinued at once. The next time, it should be undertaken less rapidly or vigorously.

Good conditioning results apparently are obtained only if larger muscle groups are exercised for at least a half hour three times a week. Loss of conditioning occurs quickly if a sedentary life-style is resumed.

Exercise in too hot, too humid, or too cold weather, after meals, after severe emotional upset, immediately after or during an illness, or at high altitudes should be avoided because it may lead to excessive strain for the heart and possible complications.

Under some circumstances, your physician may recommend

an exercise stress test prior to starting your program in order to establish the amount of exercise suitable for your heart.

SMOKING AS A RISK FACTOR

Just How Much of a Risk Is Smoking?

Each year 300,000 Americans die prematurely from the effects of smoking, according to the American Lung Association. Millions more live on with overstrained hearts and crippled lungs.

Cigarette smoking, as you may well have heard before, is a major cause of lung cancer, chronic bronchitis, and emphysema. Of all primary lung cancer cases—that is, lung cancers originating in the lungs and not spreading there from elsewhere in the body—95 percent occur in people who smoke cigarettes.

What Is the Risk in Terms of the Heart?

To some extent, it has been overshadowed by the risk of lung disease. But smoking stacks up as an important factor in coronary heart disease, and, as such, has been getting increasing attention in recent years.

Actually, the first indication of smoking's importance in heart and blood vessel disease came early in this century, with the recognition of a disease called Buerger's disease that affects small arteries and veins in the extremities, reducing blood flow. If uncontrolled, it may produce gangrene and require amputation. When the disease was first recognized, it became apparent that its victims benefited when they stopped smoking.

About the time of World War II, there was a suggestion of a link between smoking and heart disease when electrocardiograms of seemingly healthy men began to reveal a higher rate of abnormal readings among smokers than nonsmokers.

Then came a major United States study on the incidence of lung cancer among smokers, covering more than 180,000 men. The same study also demonstrated a relationship between smoking and heart disease, the death rate from coronary heart disease being more than twice as high for smokers of one pack or more daily as for nonsmokers.

There have been many studies since. In the Framingham Study, the heart attack risk was nearly double in heavy cigarette smokers; there was a threefold excess of sudden deaths among smokers compared with nonsmokers, and the sudden death risk in heavy smokers was as much as five times greater.

But Why? What Does Smoking Do?

A single cigarette can speed up heartbeat, increase blood pressure, alter the flow of blood and air in the lungs, and cause a drop in the skin temperature of extremities.

Cigarette smoke slows down the action of the cilia inside the bronchial tubes of the lungs. These tiny, rhythmically moving hairs protect the lungs by sweeping out germs, mucus, and dust. Smoke paralyzes the cilia, which allows your lungs to be more exposed to infection. In addition to irritating the breathing tubes and lungs, inhaling the hot smoke of a cigarette also damages the mouth and throat.

The lungs retain 85 to 99 percent of the compounds inhaled in cigarette smoke. The most harmful compounds are nicotine, tar, and carbon monoxide. Nicotine makes the blood vessels constrict, which then requires the heart to pump harder for blood and oxygen to circulate throughout the body. Tar, the particulate matter found in smoke, collects in the lungs and forms a brown, sticky mass containing chemicals that help cause lung cancer. Carbon monoxide decreases significantly the oxygen content of the red cells in the blood, diminishing the oxygen supply to the body. Even as nicotine increases the heart's demand for oxygen and other nutrients, carbon monoxide is decreasing the ability of the blood to supply the oxygen.

Smoking, according to a study done in Israel, also lowers the level of high-density lipoproteins, which may have a protective effect against atherosclerosis, and it is particularly dangerous for young women on birth control pills.

The latest figures indicate that the death rate from coronary heart disease is 70 percent higher for men smokers than for men nonsmokers. Women between the ages of forty-five and fifty-four who are heavy smokers have a death rate from heart disease twice that of women who do not smoke.

What About Pipes and Cigars?

Smoking cigars or a pipe is not free of other risk, such as oral cancer, but there is less risk of heart disease than with cigarette smoking. A possible reason is that a cigar smoker usually does not inhale and even if he does he seldom inhales as deeply as a cigarette smoker. This is also true for the pipe smoker, who in addition may spend somewhat less time smoking because of the time spent packing and tamping and lighting and relighting the pipe.

How Can I Go About Breaking the Habit? (I've Tried Unsuccessfully Before)

Even if your previous efforts didn't work out, you may well succeed now. The U.S. Public Health Service has estimated that 21 million Americans have given up cigarette smoking.

You will find more and more physicians interested in helping patients to break the habit. Many physicians, having done so themselves, know the ropes, and can provide helpful advice and suggestions.

Hypnosis seems to help some, though not all, who want to give up smoking. Some physicians make use of it as a help for some patients.

Group sessions also help some people. Various organizations conduct group sessions in many communities. For example, the Seventh-Day Adventists have sponsored group programs in many areas—often intensive programs carried out during five consecutive evening sessions.

The New York City Health Department has used group-session programs, with encouraging results for hundreds of people. The programs start with a lecture to assure smokers that they have the ability to eliminate the habit and that doing so can be rewarding. Each is asked to draw up a list of reasons for quitting and to keep a daily smoking record, noting time, activities, and feelings associated with each cigarette so as to better understand factors associated with the smoking habit and help break into the unconscious reflex aspects.

Smokers then meet in groups of fifteen twice a week for four weeks, then once a week for another four weeks. In the sessions, smokers can choose sudden or gradual withdrawal and help each other.

Are There Ways I Can Break the Habit on My Own?

You may well be able to do so.

Exercise may be one aid; it is for many. It has been observed that when people exercise more, they tend to smoke less.

Some smokers have found it best to pick a day on which to stop cold. Others reduce smoking gradually, using some definite schedule, such as setting up certain hours during which they will not smoke and gradually increasing the nonsmoking periods.

Some have found that they do best by simply promising themselves that they will stop for just one day at a time. When they achieve the one day of no smoking, they promise themselves another such day. And go on from day to day. It works for some.

The American Cancer Society has gathered useful suggestions from many experimental stop-smoking projects and from psychologists and medical and health authorities and published them in a pamphlet, "If You Want to Give Up Cigarettes." The pamphlet, with its specific advice and details, is reproduced in part in Appendix G.

STRESS AS A RISK FACTOR

How Much of a Factor in Heart Attacks Is Stress?

Investigators have found that emotional stress may play a role, but it's important to understand that what they are talking about is prolonged excessive stress.

Not all stress is bad. Life is full of stress. Stress occurs when you play a game of tennis or watch a motion picture or TV thriller.

It was Dr. Hans Selye who in 1950 introduced the whole concept of stress. Dr. Selye, who is director of the University of Montreal's Institute of Experimental Medicine and Surgery, has defined stress as "the nonspecific response of the body to any demand made upon it."

Of course, the body responds to specific stimuli in specific ways. If you're cold, for example, you may shiver; if you're hot, you may sweat. But in addition there is always a biologic stress reaction, the same kind of response to things as different as a painful burn or news that you have won a sweepstakes.

In the stress reaction, the adrenal glands secrete adrenaline and other hormones, mustering body energies. The reaction is basically defensive. But, as Dr. Selye has pointed out, if it is excessive or otherwise faulty it may cause disease. He writes:

> If a blow breaks a bone, if a knife penetrates the skin, the resulting damage is due to the injurious agent itself. However, many diseases have no identifiable single cause and can be produced by anything to which our stress mechanism responds inappropriately. Among the best-known diseases of adaptation are gastrointestinal ulcers, high blood pressure, cardiac (heart) accidents, allergies, and many types of mental derangements.
>
> An example will explain in principle how diseases can be produced indirectly, by our inappropriate adaptive reactions. If you meet a drunk who showers you with insults, nothing will happen if you go past and ignore him. But, if you respond, you may start a fight and get hurt, not only by the drunk but also by your own emotional reactions which increase your blood pressure, accelerate your pulse, and change the entire biochemistry of your body in a dangerous manner.

Stress as a factor in disease, including heart disease, as indicated, usually bulks up as important not necessarily on the basis of one episode or even half a dozen or a dozen episodes but rather when it is prolonged and great.

What Work Would Cause Dangerous Stress?

Some years ago, a study of one hundred young coronary patients found that at the time of their heart attacks ninety-one of these men were holding down two jobs, working more than 60 hours a week, or experiencing unusual fear, insecurity, discontent, frustration, restlessness, or feelings of inadequacy in connection with their work.

In another study, questionnaires were sent to more than twelve thousand professional people in fourteen occupational groups to compare the prevalence of coronary disease in various job categories, and among those surveyed were physicians, dentists, and lawyers in general practice and in specialties.

Coronary heart disease was found to be three times more frequent among general medical practitioners, for example, than among such specialists as dermatologists, who presumably have more regular hours and, by the nature of their work, may face less stressful situations. Similarly, trial lawyers were more prone to coronary disease than patent attorneys, whose work may be less stressful.

But Is It All a Matter of the Kind of Job?

No. If that were the case, you might reasonably think that the higher the position, the greater the stress. There is, in fact, a false stereotype that pictures the business executive as a hard-driving, pressure-ridden person with great propensity for ulcers and early heart attacks.

A large-scale study covered 270,000 men employed by the Bell System operating companies. These were men of different jobs, levels of achievement, and education. The study failed to find that men with great responsibility had any more risk of heart attack than those with lesser responsibility. Actually, the study found that those with college educations and those successful in achieving their goals had fewer heart attacks than the less educated or less successful. Apparently the less educated were less prepared and had to work harder and under greater stress to achieve and hold their jobs.

It appears that personality enters into the picture—personality as it determines how one reacts to stress and even how one may impose stresses on oneself.

Some years ago a distinguished investigator observed that the coronary-prone individual is like the mythological Sisyphus, who passed the time in hell pushing a large rock up a steep hill and never quite getting it there. The coronary disease candidate, it was noted, is a person who not only meets a challenge by putting out extra effort but takes little satisfaction from his or her accomplishments.

More recently, two San Francisco physicians have emphasized the importance of personality and behavior in coronary heart disease. They consider that there are two major types of personality, types A and B, with type A being the coronary-prone.

How Can I Tell If I Am a Type-A Person?

The investigators have suggested that if a person with type-A behavior had to wear an emblem to indicate his or her personality it might well be a clenched fist holding a stopwatch.

The type-A person is aggressive, ambitious, and competitive, has intense drive, must get things done, and almost habitually is pitted against the clock.

Type-A people generally have little time to "waste" on the beauties of life, such as love, travel, rest, vacation, literature, and art. They may have no time for friendships and are often impatient, sometimes hostile. They try to finish every task as soon as possible, want to do everything by themselves, and will tackle increasingly larger work loads, work which frequently is beyond their capacity.

They love competing with fellow workers and would much prefer to have their associates' respect rather than affection. Let anyone delay or interfere with something they want to do and their hostility may become apparent in voice and even on the face. Even with their own children, if they play games with them, they tend to play to win.

These are some of the characteristics of the type-A personality, the type with greater tendency to heart disease.

People with type-B personality, on the other hand, may be just as serious but are much more easygoing, don't feel driven by time, and can enjoy leisure.

Most of us are mixtures, with characteristics of both types, but usually one or the other predominates in varying degrees.

The type-A personality is often demanded by technologically industrialized societies, which may suggest something about the epidemic proportions of heart disease in the United States today.

How Does Type-A Behavior Relate to Heart Disease?

In one early study, the San Francisco investigators had a group of lay people choose from among their friends those who seemed to them to be typical type-A people. They furnished the names of 83 men. Another group was then asked to name 83 men who seemed most typical of type B. When all the men subsequently were thoroughly examined, 23 of the 83 type-A men (28 percent) had symptoms or electrocardiographic indications of coronary heart disease. In contrast, only 3 type-B men (4 percent) showed any evidence of heart disease.

That, of course, doesn't mean that any type-A person will have seven times as much risk of coronary heart disease as a type-B person. The eighty-three men in each category were extremes of the types. But the results did suggest to the investigators that people with type-A behavior are relatively prone to heart disease and those with type-B are less so.

The same kind of study was carried out for women. Again, groups of lay people chose from among their friends and acquaintances 125 women they considered to fit the type-A category and 132 who seemed to fit the type-B. Most of the type-A women worked in industry or in professional jobs; most of the type-B were housewives. The type-A women had more coronary heart disease (19 percent) than did the type-B women (4 percent).

These, of course, were retrospective studies, that is, they dealt with men and women who had one or the other kind of personality and behavior pattern and who either already had or did not have heart disease. And they indicated that heart disease was four to seven times more common in those with type-A than in those with type-B behavior. But they didn't prove that anyone with type-A behavior who had no heart disease would be more apt to develop it in the future than anyone with type-B behavior.

So, in a later study supported by the National Institutes of Health, the investigators picked 3,500 men ranging in age from thirty-nine to fifty-nine, all without any indication of heart disease.

They were examined, carefully interviewed, and classified as type A or type B. In the study, a prospective one, the men have been followed continuously. Even by the end of four years, 52 had developed a first heart attack and 18 others had experienced a first attack of angina pectoris, indicating coronary heart disease.

The incidence of the disease was three times greater among the type-A than among the type-B men. Several years later, when 257 of the men had developed coronary heart disease, 70 percent of them proved to be type A.

Are There Specific Effects of Type-A Behavior?

The investigators sought to determine whether the behavior pattern, or some aspect of it, such as working under deadlines, might affect blood cholesterol levels. They got the cooperation of a group of accountants who agreed to take cholesterol-measuring blood tests twice a month for six months.

The accountants showed no particularly well-developed type-A or B patterns under normal circumstances. But when they came under special stress just before the April tax deadlines, their blood tests showed cholesterol levels that were significantly higher than at other times.

During the six months of testing, some of the men experienced personal stressful situations that they reported to be more severe than tax-deadline stresses. When blood cholesterol was checked at such times, it was markedly higher than at other times.

When cholesterol levels were checked in women, the levels in type-A women proved to be considerably higher on the average than those in type-B women.

It also appears from the research that extreme type-A men and women tend to smoke more cigarettes per day than Bs and also to find less time and have less inclination to exercise or engage in recreational physical activity.

Can I Eliminate the Type-A Risk Factor?

Probably yes. It will not be easy, but with a lot of determination and conscious decisions, it can be done.

You must bear in mind that you might not be as "successful" in your various business and other undertakings as you might be with continued type-A behavior, and you should be prepared to accept that.

On the other hand, you may well be able to get along better with those you love and with people in general. You may be able to establish and develop more friendships, and you may begin to enjoy life more on a day-to-day basis.

The decision to change type-A personality before you may develop heart disease is, in a sense, entirely yours to make.

After you have a heart attack or develop heart disease, the question becomes more acute. Quite simply, continuing type-A behavior may substantially shorten your life. Heart disease is serious, and type-A behavior may aggravate it. At this point, therefore, the choice becomes a medical as well as personal one.

You may need and benefit from counseling and guidance by your physician. Your physician may refer you to a psychiatrist. Psychiatric consultation—it doesn't by any means have to be a matter of years of sessions on a couch—may be most helpful after relatively brief exploration of your life-style and problems. Or you may want to talk with a clergyman of your faith.

What it comes down to in the end is a taking stock of your life-style. You should realistically assess your capabilities and just what it is you want out of life for yourself and for your family. Being realistic is very important. Do not set goals that are beyond your capability or goals that will require every ounce of your capability to achieve.

Do not envy people who may be more capable in some specific area than you are. You may be more capable in another than they are. Accept the fact that you excel in certain matters and not in others.

Learn that you do not have to do everything yourself, that you can delegate some responsibility and some tasks to others. Learn to say no when you are asked to accept excessive new responsibilities.

Never be afraid that others will outshine and surpass you. Don't worry if, perhaps, younger people who may be physically stronger or who may have more formal education, and who may be hard-driving A types, excel you. They may regret their aggressive type-A behavior later.

Learn to set aside adequate time for each task. Avoid deadlines as much as possible, and certainly those that are self-imposed. Leave more time for appointments and more time to rest and refresh yourself between every few appointments.

Do not let work intrude on all other aspects of your life. Take time out to make new friends and to enjoy old ones. Take time to enjoy your family. Enjoy leisure, art, literature, nature, walks, or simply free time for reflection. Don't feel that you always have to be occupied with something. You do not have to use all your time productively. You must have some leisure time to enjoy yourself.

Realize that you can't finish everything in a day—nor, indeed, in a lifetime. Enjoy every day for its own sake.

The possibility of your own death will probably occur to you. Do not be afraid to die. This may be difficult, since many of us were trained from childhood to fear death. But it is important that you accept your own mortality and realize that all people, indeed all living beings, one day will stop living.

Realize that life is a gift. Enjoy it and make the most of it. Although someday your life must end, you can approach that day—which will probably occur in the more distant future than you think—with the fulfilling knowledge that you have lived in the best way you knew how.

Learn that each age has its own virtues and rewards. Learn what those are. You should not try to live the life of a teenager when you are over fifty. On the other hand, you should take comfort in the knowledge that it is not all downhill. Remember the successes of your earlier years and exercise the virtues of wisdom, reflection, and contentment.

These are all important for your years ahead. It is important that you be content and not fear death, because if you have heart disease, such anxieties can increase the chances of a heart attack.

Remember that each of us in our own way continues to be part of our children, friends, colleagues, and co-workers, and this is the way it has been since time immemorial.

HIGH URIC-ACID LEVELS (GOUT) AS A RISK FACTOR

Is It Really a Fact That Gout Increases the Risk of Coronary Heart Disease?

Yes, there does seem to be increased risk. The Framingham Study has produced evidence that there is a 1.6 times increase in risk of coronary heart disease associated with elevated uric-acid levels.

Is Gout a Pain in the Toe?

Actually, gout doesn't have to involve a pain in a toe, although the big toe is the classical site of attack. Gout can be a pain in any joint, or it may involve no pain at all.

Gout is an inherited disorder, largely but not entirely confined to men, in which uric-acid levels in the blood are elevated.

In gout, the body is unable to properly handle certain important compounds, called purines, which occur in a variety of foods and are also normally formed in the body. As a result of that inability, uric acid—which is a breakdown product of purines—builds up in the blood.

Sometimes the excess uric acid may be deposited in a joint, producing an inflammatory reaction that leads to severe pain, swelling, and redness. Not infrequently, the uric-acid level may be elevated without producing symptoms of any kind. The elevation may then be discovered during a medical checkup when a routine blood test for uric acid is ordered.

Whether or not symptoms occur, elevated uric-acid levels, as the Framingham Study has indicated, are associated with increased risk of coronary heart disease. Exactly how this occurs is not understood. It has been proposed but not proven that high concentrations of uric acid in the blood may in some manner make the inner walls of the coronary arteries susceptible to damage by cholesterol.

What Can Be Done About Gout or Elevated Uric-Acid Levels?

When it comes to a gout attack itself, an old drug called colchicine—an extract of the meadow saffron, an herb—is a specific for treatment. It usually stops an attack within twenty-four hours.

Another class of drugs can promote the elimination of excess uric acid through the kidneys. One is probenecid, first put to use during World War II when penicillin was newly discovered and in short supply. Probenecid was found to be a penicillin "extender"—capable of making small amounts of the antibiotic go further in treatment. Later, it proved a help with gout and with elevated uric-acid levels. Probenecid now is often used in small daily doses, by itself or in combination with colchicine, to lower uric-acid levels and prevent many gout attacks. Sulfinpyrazone is another useful drug that acts much like probenecid.

A newer agent, allopurinol, acts to block the working of an enzyme that converts compounds into uric acid. By reducing production of uric acid, it reduces uric-acid levels in the blood. It also seems to stimulate the breakdown and excretion of uric-acid deposits that may already have accumulated in the body.

If your uric-acid levels are elevated, whether or not you have experienced any gout attacks with joint pain, your physician may think it wise to prescribe suitable medication.

DIABETES AS A RISK FACTOR

What's the Significance of Diabetes in Heart Disease?

Diabetes can be a very subtle disease, as well as a relatively common one. It's known to affect millions of Americans, including several million who are not even aware they have it.

The Framingham Study has found that among men ages thirty to fifty-nine initially free of coronary heart disease, diabetics developed 1.4 times the amount of heart disease as did nondiabetics—and the incidence of heart disease in diabetic women was 2.5 times greater than in those who were nondiabetic. The study also determined that the risk of death from coronary heart disease is 2.3 times higher in diabetic men and 5.7 times higher in diabetic women.

Researchers have found that cholesterol levels tend to be higher in diabetics than in nondiabetics, that high blood pressure is nearly twice as frequent, and that about four of every five newly discovered adult diabetics are overweight.

There have been other studies showing the relationship between diabetes and heart disease. At the Joslin Clinic in Boston, a famed diabetes research and treatment center, 46.5 percent of deaths in diabetics have been found to be caused by coronary heart disease.

To check on factors influencing health, University of Michigan medical researchers persuaded 8,600 residents of Tecumseh, Michigan, nine tenths of the community, to undergo various tests. They found a high frequency of coronary disease among the diabetics in the population and they also found that people with heart disease tended to have diabetes. It appeared that many with coronary disease could be mild diabetics in whom the coronary problem could overshadow the sugar-handling problem of diabetes.

Why Might I Have Diabetes Without Knowing It?

Diabetes doesn't necessarily signal its presence with unmistakable pain or clear-cut early warning signs. In the early stages or in a mild case of diabetes, the victim may feel nothing more than listlessness, if that. Later, there may be thirst, urinary frequency, loss of weight despite good appetite, itching particularly of the genital area in women, and recurrent skin infections.

In diabetes, the body is unable to handle sugar properly—either because of lack of insulin or ineffective use of the hormone.

Normally, all carbohydrates—starches and sugars—are converted in the body to a type of sugar called glucose. Ultimately, much of protein food is also turned into glucose. It is glucose that travels by way of the blood to all tissues to be used to produce energy.

In severe diabetes, because of the inability to handle glucose, it accumulates in the blood. When it builds to high enough levels—about 180 milligrams or more of glucose for every 100 milliliters of blood—the glucose begins to spill over into the urine. It takes water with it and large amounts of urine are passed, leading to great thirst. If the diabetes is not controlled, the body, unable to use sugar, then uses fats. But the breakdown of large amounts of fats can lead to accumulation of acid products in the blood. The victim may gasp for breath, and if the condition is still not corrected shock and death may follow.

But, as I have indicated, with mild diabetes, the symptoms may be nonexistent for long periods or so mild that unless there are routine checks to discover diabetes, advanced complications—such as vision and nerve difficulties, boils, and coronary heart disease—may be the first symptoms of concern.

Who Is Likely to Get Diabetes?

Although diabetes tends to run in families, anybody can get it at any age.

It affects some children. More often, it appears later in life, and is called adult-onset diabetes. Most of those who develop diabetes as adults are obese.

What Can Be Done About It?

Usually, a child with diabetes needs insulin. His or her pancreas does not produce enough of the hormone.

In adult-onset diabetes, on the other hand, insulin production is commonly adequate but the insulin is not effectively used. Therefore, in many adult-onset cases, diet alone is sufficient to overcome the problem, restoring blood-sugar levels to normal. In other adults, insulin or oral hypoglycemics—drugs that can be taken by mouth to lower blood-sugar levels—may be used.

Will Treatment for Diabetes Insure Against Coronary Heart Disease?

No, since other risk factors also may be present and need control.

There has also been a school of medicine which has held that treatment for diabetes does not necessarily eliminate diabetes itself as a risk factor in heart disease—that, even with control, somehow diabetes may still contribute to the development of atherosclerosis.

But recent evidence has convinced the American Diabetes Association that tight control of diabetes, careful attention to maintaining blood glucose at normal levels, may in fact reduce the risk of blood vessel disturbances.

If it should turn out that you have diabetes, even quite mild diabetes, your physician may well want to make certain that it is well controlled. He or she may accomplish that with your cooperation, by diet and weight control. If necessary, medication may be prescribed.

DRINKING WATER
AND OTHER POSSIBLE RISK FACTORS

Can the Kind of Water I Drink Have an Effect on My Heart?

Various studies suggesting this possibility generally have shown an inverse correlation between hard water and heart disease—that is, the harder the water, the less the incidence of heart disease. A distinguished British epidemiologist has presented evidence correlating water hardness and heart disease mortality in regions throughout England and Wales. Other studies elsewhere have suggested similar correlation.

In the British studies, covering sixty-one county boroughs with populations of eighty thousand or more, the harder the drinking water, the lower the death rate in middle age and early old age. The relationship seemed to hold particularly true for heart and blood vessel diseases.

What Benefits Could Hard Water Have?

The question is a complex one, and much remains to be learned.

Water gets its hardness from the calcium and magnesium it contains; the more of these two elements, the harder water is. One of many suggestions is that blood cholesterol levels may be reduced by hard water, possibly because calcium and magnesium may combine with saturated fats in foods and so reduce the body's assimilation of such fats.

Another theory blames soft water for being a possible factor in heart disease, not because of its lower content of calcium and magnesium but because of its higher content of cadmium.

One researcher believes that while hard water lays down a protective lime coating in water pipes, soft water does not. Instead, he considers that soft water picks up some carbon dioxide and becomes slightly acid, and, thanks to the acidity, it dissolves out and picks up cadmium, copper, lead, and other metals from pipes. He feels that cadmium in particular is a key factor in the development of both high blood pressure and atherosclerosis. If cadmium is an important factor, it may not be because of soft water alone. Cadmium may enter the water supply through industrial pollution.

For practical purposes, studies of the relationship of drinking water to heart disease have just begun. I tend to think that it would be premature at this time to go to any great lengths to artificially harden your water if you live in a soft-water area.

What About the Possible Risk in Drinking Water That Is High in Salt?

Here we are on well-established ground.

A water supply that is high in sodium will tend to make you retain water and, in so doing, may elevate your blood pressure and increase the chance of congestive heart failure if you already have heart disease.

So for the same reason that you should stay away from excess salt in your diet, you should also stay away from sodium-rich waters.

The sodium content of the water in your area can usually be obtained from your local department of health. If the water is high in sodium, then a change to another form of drinking water may be indicated. It should be noted that bottled carbonated drinks often contain large amounts of sodium.

Is It True That a Lack of Chromium in Refined Foods May Be a Factor?

Studies have suggested that this may be so.

If chromium is eliminated completely from the diets of rats, within a few months 80 percent develop sugary urine, indicative of a diabetic state.

Human autopsy studies have revealed that the amount of chromium in tissues declines as people get older. As compared with newborns, for example, adults have only one third the chromium level.

Research also indicates that when we eat carbohydrates—both sugar and starches—the sugar level in the blood rises and in response the pancreas sends an increased supply of insulin into the blood. At the same time, chromium is mobilized from body stores and moves into the blood to work with the insulin in handling the sugar. When the job is done, the chromium in the blood circulates to the kidneys where about 20 percent of it is excreted in the urine.

As long as the sugar and starch in the diet contain adequate chromium, enough of the metal can be absorbed to make up for the losses in the urine and there is no net loss. But if the sugar or starch or both contain very little chromium, there is a net loss from the body and chromium stores are depleted more and more over a period of time.

The fact is that the refined sugar and starch most commonly used in our diet are very low in chromium. Raw sugar has a rich supply, some 36 micrograms per 150 grams. But refined white sugar contains only 3 to 4 micrograms per 150 grams.

White flour is also chromium deficient. While whole wheat flour contains 175 micrograms per 100 grams, refined white flour contains only 23. So white flour may cause depletion of body chromium just as refined sugar does.

It therefore appears that the typical diet in Western nations, with so many calories coming from refined sugar and refined flour, could hardly have been better designed to provide as little chromium as possible and to deplete body stores of it by not replacing urinary losses.

This could be one reason that it may pay to reduce excessive sugar intake and make greater use of unrefined carbohydrates—whole wheat bread in place of a diet all of refined white bread, whole meal flour to replace at least some of the refined white flour used at home in preparing various dishes.

What Does All This About Risk Factors Add Up to for Me?

Virtually all diseases are complex. Many factors enter into them. Certainly that is true of coronary heart disease.

Undoubtedly, we have much yet to learn about the heart problem. But we have also learned a lot. Remember that it wasn't so long ago when atherosclerosis with its deadly effects was considered something that was inevitable with aging and therefore not capable of being fought effectively.

We know much better than that now. We can make inroads against it. Considering what we know now about risk factors, it makes sense to reduce or eliminate them.

It is highly likely that you will benefit to some degree—and quite possibly to a great degree—by countering those risk factors that apply in your particular case: by following your physician's advice on using diet, and if necessary medication, to reduce elevated blood fat levels, by avoiding cigarette smoking, by exercising regularly as your physician may prescribe, by controlling your weight, by controlling any disorder you may have such as high blood pressure, diabetes, or high uric-acid levels that may favor the development or progression of atherosclerosis, and by reducing stress as much as possible.

If you follow these guidelines and comply faithfully with your physician's advice, there is a good chance that your heart disease may remain well controlled and that a heart attack may never occur or recur. Do what you are supposed to do and then enjoy life without being constantly tortured and obsessed by a fear of death. Discussion with your family will help them also to adopt the same attitude and allow you to live a much happier and probably longer life.

6

Tests for the Heart: What They Are, What They Help Reveal

Everyone who has or is suspected of having coronary heart disease will be examined and given tests, most if not all of which may be mysterious to the patient. They need not be. In this chapter, I answer questions you may have about the procedures—including electrocardiography, echocardiography, nuclear scanning, catheterization, blood tests, and others—when and why they may be used, what they can show, and what it's like for the patient going through them.

Why Is the Pulse Taken?

It's common for physicians to begin a physical examination by taking the pulse. Usually the pulse rate is the same as the heart rate although occasionally, with a very rapid or irregular heartbeat, for example, there may be some difference between the two. This difference is called a pulse deficit.

A normal pulse rate generally ranges from 60 to 80 beats a minute, although it may go higher in some normal people. The rate can vary considerably not only from one person to another but at different times in the same person. It will go up, for example, with exercise or emotional stress, and with fever.

But the rate also increases when blood pressure is high and when hyperthyroidism, or overfunctioning of the thyroid gland, is present. It also increases with congestive heart failure, a condition in which the heart because of underlying disease has lost some of its pumping efficiency, resulting in a tendency for fluids to accumulate in body tissues. Trying to make up for its lost pumping efficiency, the heart then may beat faster.

On the other hand, in some heart disorders and in hypothyroidism, or underfunctioning of the thyroid gland, the heart and pulse rates often slow down.

So your physician can get much information about your heart and its functioning, as well as about the possibility of other disease being present, from the pulse—not only its rate but also its strength and rhythm.

Why Do Physicians so Often Repeat Blood Pressure Measurements Even During the Same Visit?

To try to get a true picture of what the pressure is. Having blood pressure taken arouses some anxiety, conscious or not, in many people—and hence the pressure goes up. So to try to eliminate the anxiety factor and get an accurate reading, the physician may repeat the measurement several times.

Why Do Physicians Sometimes Take Blood Pressure Readings in the Legs as Well as the Arms?

A relatively rare cause of high blood pressure is coarctation, or narrowing, of a section of the aorta, the body's trunkline artery from which other arteries branch off.

Because the narrowing obstructs the flow of blood, pressure increases. Usually the narrowing occurs at a point just beyond where arteries carrying blood to the head and arms branch off. And the blood pressure rise occurs in those vessels because they are ahead of the obstruction and not in the vessels leading to the legs.

So if a physician finds blood pressure elevated when taken in the arms and has any reason to suspect that coarctation may be present, he or she will take a reading of pressure in the legs. If that pressure is lower than the arm pressure, it helps to confirm the suspicion. Coarctation is curable by surgery.

Tests for the Heart

Why Are Eyes Examined When the Problem Is with the Heart?

It's not to evaluate vision, but by using an instrument called an ophthalmoscope the physician can see through the pupils of the eyes and view the retina and its blood vessels. Those vessels are tinier than any others that can be seen readily elsewhere in the body and their condition can provide an indication of the presence or absence of artery disease.

Such an examination can also be valuable, when a patient has high blood pressure, in determining how long the elevated pressure has been present before detection by seeing how those delicate vessels may or may not have been affected.

What's the Purpose of Examining Virtually the Whole Body?

For one thing, the physician can note any swelling, especially in the legs, that may indicate excess fluid accumulation, which may be indicative of heart disease.

The skin can often provide clues. If it is pale and cold when the environmental temperature is comfortable, it may sometimes indicate that the heart is not pumping properly.

If the skin is unusually warm when the environmental temperature is comfortable, it may be the result of excessive thyroid functioning or possibly some abnormal blood vessel connections.

What Can Feeling the Chest Reveal?

Feeling the chest with the fingers is called palpation. It can sometimes provide a clue. For example, trained fingers can detect a kind of pulsation called the apex beat in the space between the fifth and sixth ribs. The pulsation is normally weak, and if it should be exaggerated it may indicate a heart problem, such as increased size of the left ventricle, or pumping chamber, of the heart.

What Can the Stethoscope Reveal?

Using the stethoscope to listen to the heart—called *auscultation*—may provide important information.

When the heart contracts, it produces first a "lubb" sound and then a "dup" sound. If these sounds deviate from normal, it suggests a heart problem and can be helpful in diagnosis.

As you probably know, murmurs can be detected through the stethoscope. A murmur is a noise that may occur when there are structural abnormalities in the heart or peculiar kinds of blood flow through the heart's chambers. An experienced physician can often identify the particular problem from the timing, intensity, and characteristics of the murmur.

Let me hasten to add that parents are often confused about murmurs in children. Many murmurs are innocent, produced by slight peculiarities that are not significant and do not indicate heart problems of any kind.

What's the Value of an Electrocardiogram?

An electrocardiogram—also known as an EKG or ECG—is an invaluable tool for a trained physician in diagnosing conditions affecting the heart.

When any muscle of the body moves, it produces small electrical currents. The heart is one of the most powerful of body muscles and it produces a rhythmic output of electrical current.

The electrocardiograph is a machine that painlessly detects and amplifies the heart's currents and traces them onto a strip of paper to produce the record called the electrocardiogram. The currents are carried to the electrocardiograph through wires from small metal plates that are placed on the skin of arms, legs, and chest with a special paste used to help assure conduction of the currents.

Electrocardiograms of normal hearts are reasonably characteristic. If there is a heart abnormality, the electrocardiogram may reveal abnormal tracings.

Abnormal tracings do not always mean that the heart is abnormal. Anxiety, fear, heavy breathing, drinking ice water, smoking, use of some drugs, and certain nonheart illnesses may make an electrocardiogram deviate from normal.

But, with due regard to such factors, an experienced physician can get a good picture of what is going on in the heart from the electrocardiogram, especially when other tests and thorough clinical examination and history are also considered.

What Heart Disturbances Does an ECG Help Diagnose?

As carefully interpreted by a skilled physician, the ECG can reveal certain heart rhythm disturbances, inadequate supply of oxygen reaching the heart muscle, and congenital or acquired heart disturbances.

It helps to diagnose a heart attack.

It can indicate shortages or excesses of certain elements in the blood, such as calcium and potassium.

Sometimes it helps to indicate the presence of a blood clot in a lung, underactivity of the thyroid gland, or inflammation of the pericardium, which is the sac surrounding the heart.

In addition to its value in diagnosis, the ECG can be of vital importance in the coronary care unit when a patient has had a heart attack or may be experiencing one.

When the heart stops or fibrillates, the electrocardiogram indicates this fact and cardiac resuscitation can be started immediately. In the coronary care unit, nurses carefully monitor heart rhythms on a televisionlike screen connected to the electrocardiograph leads.

The medical staff can become aware immediately not only of heart stoppage but also of potentially dangerous rhythms as soon as they develop. The most dangerous is fibrillation, in which the ventricles of the heart may only quiver uselessly instead of pump. With prompt action, fibrillation often can be converted to normal beating. And, in fact, specially trained nurses carefully monitor for abnormal rhythms that may precede fibrillation so that prompt action can be taken to forestall the development of fibrillation.

Incidentally, it takes great experience to properly interpret the electrocardiogram on the TV screen. Many harmless shape and rhythm changes can result from the patient's movements, breathing, or even to loose leads. It is therefore wise, as I indicated earlier, for the patient not to watch the screen of the monitor so as to avoid unfounded apprehension and fear.

What's the Purpose of a Portable Heart Monitor?

Rhythm disturbances of the heart are not always continuous; some may be intermittent, and a regular diagnostic electrocardiogram may miss them since they are brief.

If there is reason to suspect the existence of such disturbances, a Holter ECG is used to detect them. A special instrument is attached to the standard ECG leads taped to the chest and the patient can carry it unobtrusively by an over-the-shoulder strap during normal activities at home, at work, and even during many recreational activities.

Instead of being transferred directly to a piece of paper, the electrical impulses from the heart are recorded on magnetic tape in the instrument. The patient may wear it over a period of eight to twenty-four hours and all during that time the electrical impulses from the heart are being recorded.

Afterward, the tape recording can be played back by the physician on a special unit called a scanner in about forty-five minutes. Should any abnormality be noticed, a regular paper recording of this portion of the tape can easily be obtained.

The Holter ECG is valuable because it can monitor the patient's heart activity over an extended period and under varying conditions—exercising, at rest, eating, sleeping, times of mental calm, times of emotional stress.

In fact, if your physician wishes to use a Holter ECG, he or she will probably indicate that you should continue all your normal activities while wearing it, except for bathing, since water may damage the tape.

No test is infallible, of course. The Holter ECG is very helpful but occasionally, like any other test, it may fail to reveal a problem (false negative) or indicate a problem that is not actually present (false positive).

What Is a Stress Test?

A conventional ECG is taken with the patient at rest, stretched out usually on an examining table. There are some abnormalities of the heart, however, that manifest themselves only while the body is active. To discover such abnormalities, when they are suspected, a stress or exercise test may be used while an ECG is taken.

The exercise may consist of climbing three stairs for three minutes, pedaling a stationary bicycle, or walking a treadmill. The bicycle activity can gradually be made more strenuous by increasing the resistance to pedaling. And the treadmill activity can gradually be made more strenuous by increasing the speed of operation, the angle of incline, or both.

With a stress test, the physician may sometimes detect abnormalities that would not otherwise be revealed with a conventional ECG. He or she can also observe the response of the heart to measured energy expenditures and can then estimate how much activity a patient may be able to tolerate safely.

Stress ECGs should be taken with the proper equipment and medication available in case of emergency. A trained physician who is able to recognize and deal with emergencies should be present.

Because there is some risk associated with the test, even though that risk is relatively small, and because some doubt as to its value has been raised recently, it should not be performed routinely. In particular, it should not be done routinely with patients in whom the diagnosis has been established clearly without it, in patients who have highly abnormal resting electrocardiograms, in those who have had recent heart attacks, or in patients in whom angina has recently increased.

However, I have found, as have many other cardiologists, that the stress ECG has great value in carefully selected patients. It is most important to keep in mind that such a test could be falsely positive or negative. The results must be carefully evaluated in conjunction with all other clinical findings and should not be taken at face value.

What Is Echocardiography?

This is a technique of recording the echoes of ultrasonic waves—very-high-frequency sound waves that are beyond the range of hearing—when these waves are directed at areas of the heart with a high-frequency generator placed on the chest. The principle is to some extent similar to that used in sonar detection of submarines.

As the ultrasonic waves pass through the heart, they behave differently depending on such conditions as whether or not calcification is present, whether there is a blood clot or any other mass in the cavity of the heart, whether certain chambers of the heart are enlarged, whether the valves within the heart open and close properly, and whether some part of the heart is thicker than it should be.

Echocardiography is often useful in allowing visualization of features of the heart that might otherwise go unnoticed. Often, for example, an expert physician using echocardiography can detect an abnormal thickness of the cardiac septum, the wall within the heart, which may cause chest pain very similar to angina.

Such differential diagnosis allowed sometimes by echocardiography may be decisive. It may in some cases completely change the course of treatment and make it more effective. It may make other more complex tests unnecessary.

The procedure is simple, painless, no more troublesome for the patient than electrocardiography, and is considered harmless even for pregnant patients and their future offspring.

The heart is not the only organ capable of being visualized by means of ultrasound. Many other internal organs—and also the fetus during pregnancy—can be visualized.

What Is Nuclear Scanning of the Heart?

This is another technique that allows visualization of the heart. Currently, nuclear scanning is being done only in large medical centers, but it has become an important diagnostic test and promises to become even more so in the near future.

Tests for the Heart

Small amounts of a radioactive isotope material are injected into a vein. Healthy heart muscle will absorb a certain amount of the isotope. But if part of the heart muscle has been affected by a heart attack, that part will absorb a different amount.

The isotope gives off radioactivity—very small, safe amounts—and this can be registered on photographic film. The amount given off, of course, depends upon the amount absorbed. And the film record can provide a picture of healthy and damaged heart muscle. From the film, the expert can determine the size of the damaged area, its behavior at rest, and its behavior upon effort.

Except for the slight discomfort from puncturing of a vein to administer the isotope, the test does not hurt and is considered by experts to be safe. It may at times make other tests, such as catheterization of the heart, unnecessary.

What Is Heart and Coronary Artery Catheterization?

This is a procedure that allows the heart chambers, blood vessels, and course of blood flow to be seen.

The patient receives a local anesthetic and a small incision is made into a blood vessel, often in the groin area or in the crease of the elbow. Then a catheter—a long, thin, flexible plastic tube—is placed in the blood vessel and slowly guided up through the vessel and into the heart. The patient feels no significant discomfort while this is going on.

Then a chemical, which is visible on X-ray films, is injected into the catheter and soon reaches the heart. X-ray movies are then made of the heart. If the chemical is also injected into the coronary arteries, the movies can disclose whether the arteries are normal or diseased.

Blood samples can be taken through the catheter to determine how much oxygen is present in the blood in different chambers of the heart. And the pressure of the blood in different chambers of the heart can be measured directly.

A cardiac team, which may consist of a cardiologist, a heart surgeon, and a radiologist, can study the X-ray movie and can stop the film at any place for close scrutiny. They can detect alterations in the heart muscle and any obstructions that may be present in the coronary arteries. They may discover that one or both coronary arteries, or one or more branches, is obstructed, either by spasm or involuntary contraction, or by atherosclerotic deposits. And they can determine the site and extent of the obstruction.

Unfortunately, catheterization has certain drawbacks. It is expensive and requires hospitalization. Often, careful examination by a competent cardiologist, using noninvasive tests such as nuclear scanning, may make catheterization unnecessary.

Finally, catheterization is not without risk. It may sometimes cause disturbances in the heart rhythm. Rarely, it may precipitate a heart attack. Still more rarely, it may result in death.

Fortunately, in the hands of experts, catheterization has a mortality rate of 0.3 percent or less, or 3 in 1,000. When performed in the past by less experienced physicians, the mortality was much higher, reaching 4 percent or more. Experts often perform many catheterizations successfully every day.

Nevertheless, such a procedure should be carried out only if there are good reasons for doing so. It should not be done needlessly if other less expensive and less possibly risky tests tell the physician what he or she wants to know. The decision is complex and catheterization should be undertaken only on the advice of your cardiologist.

It is usually indicated before heart surgery.

Under other circumstances, in case of doubt as to the need, always obtain a second opinion. Be sure to ask the cardiologist who will perform the catheterization about his or her mortality rate and the exact expense involved. A patient should always be fully informed about the nature of the test and its risks, costs, and benefits.

Why Do I Get So Many Blood Tests in the Coronary Care Unit?

Blood tests are invaluable diagnostic tools under many circumstances, and certainly after a heart attack. They can indicate whether the mixture of oxygen and carbon dioxide in the blood is satisfactory, whether the blood is too alkaline or too acid. This test, called a blood-gas determination, makes it possible to correct any serious abnormality, should it exist.

A proper balance of electrolytes—potassium, sodium, and chloride ions—is also necessary. If there is an imbalance, a blood test can reveal it and permit ready correction.

After a heart attack, in fact, there may be many things amiss in the blood. It is important to know about them so suitable action can be taken.

A blood test may be helpful in establishing the diagnosis of a heart attack. Such a test measures the levels of certain heart enzymes that escape from a damaged heart muscle into the bloodstream. Their presence in the blood in unusually increased amounts may provide a more reliable diagnosis than the electrocardiogram alone.

Frequently, blood tests can uncover anemia and other conditions of the body that may not be otherwise detectable but need correction to improve your heart condition.

7

Heart Medications and Heart Pacemakers

What is the nature of the medical agents that may be used for treatment if you have coronary heart disease, experience anginal chest pain, or have had a heart attack? What are their purposes? What, if any, undesirable effects can they cause—and what can be done in the case of such side effects? And what are pacemakers, what do they do, when may one be needed, and how may it be inserted and maintained?

Are There Any Rules I Should Follow in Taking Medication?

Your physician has probably prescribed one or more medications for you to take. Do take them, and take them exactly as prescribed; don't try to treat yourself.

Certain medications, in order to be useful for your heart condition, must be taken regularly. You may nullify their usefulness, perhaps even run a risk, if you interrupt their use or otherwise vary it.

So follow your physician's orders precisely. Make no changes, either in dosage, frequency, or time for taking a medication. Don't stop taking a prescribed medication even if you feel well or have exhausted the prescription. Renew it at once; don't wait until your next visit to the physician. If you should lose your medications replace them immediately. Should your pharmacist refuse to replace or renew a prescription, feel free to call your physician. He or she can call the pharmacist to give his or her approval.

Why Do Undesirable Side Effects Occur? If They Occur, What Should I Do?

Generally, it is difficult to design a drug that does only one thing: going precisely to the target and achieving a desired result without having any other effects.

When a drug is introduced into the body, it may sometimes cause side effects. These may vary from person to person. In some people, there may be virtually no undesirable effects or, if any occur, they may be of minor nature and without consequence. The body's handling of a particular drug can differ from one person to another just as can the handling of some ordinary food, for example.

The upset stomach associated with aspirin is a side effect for some people but not for all. Other reactions to aspirin may be more severe. Fortunately, most of the medications that you may be taking for your heart will not have appreciable side effects.

Should you experience a side effect, don't simply discontinue medication. Call your physician promptly for advice. He or she will know whether the reaction is a serious one—demanding a change of medication—or a harmless, transient one, with the benefits to be obtained far outweighing any temporary discomfort. Perhaps a slight adjustment in the dosage will eliminate the reaction. Discuss this with your physician.

It's rare, but you may be allergic or overly sensitive to a particular drug and may get an unpleasant reaction, such as a skin rash, no matter how little you take. In that case, stop taking the medication and immediately call your physician, who can decide whether you should continue or change to a different kind of medication. Often, side effects are related to the dose of the medication and they disappear when the quantity is reduced.

Sometimes different drugs taken together may cause side effects that neither would have caused if taken alone. For example, if you are taking a drug to reduce the risk of a blood clot and take aspirin for some minor pain, the result may be severe bleeding.

So be sure to let your physician know what medications of any kind, besides those he or she has prescribed, you are taking or plan to take—even drugs that you may buy without prescription for something that may have nothing to do with the heart.

DIGITALIS

What Is Digitalis and What Does It Do?

Digitalis is an extract of the foxglove plant. It's an old drug, employed for a long time, and still one of the most useful medications for heart disease.

It has two principal actions which make it valuable. First, its kind of tonic effect on the heart helps the heart muscle to make better use of energy, increases its efficiency, and enables the heart to pump more blood with each beat. Second, digitalis can help overcome certain disturbances of heart rhythm. When the heart's ventricles, or pumping chambers, are contracting excessively and inefficiently, it can slow down and regularize the contraction rate, often with dramatic improvement in a patient's condition.

Digitalis may be used under various circumstances. And I should emphasize that, contrary to the impression of some patients, its use doesn't necessarily mean that there is irreversible damage to the heart.

It may be used, for example, for congestive heart failure, when large amounts of fluids have collected in the body because of poor pumping efficiency of the heart. It can lead to the elimination of excess fluid as it improves pumping efficiency and may, after a time, even allow the heart in some cases to regain virtually normal function.

Digitalis may also be used for someone who has a rapid heartbeat even though no organic disease is present. And it may be used to help prevent heart failure in patients with heart disease who must undergo a stressful situation such as surgery.

Are There Various Forms of Digitalis?

Yes. Digitalis is prescribed as digoxin, digitoxin, Gitaligin, or—in its older form—as digitalis leaf.

Digoxin is the form most commonly used now. It usually comes in yellow tablets of 0.125 milligrams, white tablets of 0.25 milligrams, and green tablets of 0.5 milligrams. Digoxin has the advantage of rapid action. When necessary, it can also be given by injection.

Digitoxin, the other form in common use, takes longer to act, remains in the body longer, and is equally effective.

Is Proper Dosage Important?

Very much so.

The dosage of digitalis prescribed for you will depend, for one thing, on your age and weight. A smaller dosage is usually used for older patients and those small in stature and light in weight.

It will depend, too, on many other factors, such as the functioning of your kidneys, liver, heart, and thyroid, your levels of magnesium, calcium, and potassium, and on the ability of your body to absorb the drug.

Less digitalis is tolerated when heart, thyroid, kidney, or liver function is markedly decreased, if potassium or magnesium levels are decreased, or if the calcium level is increased. In all these cases the dosage must be decreased from the usual level.

Digitalis should be administered under close medical supervision, particularly if the patient is on a strict low-salt diet or is taking diuretics (see page 155), which cause a larger excretion of sodium and potassium in the urine. Most antacids should not be taken within six hours of digitalis administration because they hinder absorption of the drug by the body. Digitalis should not be taken on an empty stomach.

Your physician can monitor the dose of digitalis by taking a sample of your blood and determining the level of the drug in it. This test is usually performed not less than eight hours after the last dose. It is a helpful but not always definitive test and so has to be interpreted in terms of your total clinical picture.

The dosage of digitalis may be high during the first day or two of its use. You are then being given what is called the "digitalization dose." Once you are "digitalized" properly, a smaller maintenance dose is taken once or twice a day to replace the loss through excretion.

Under no circumstances should you discontinue digitalis or change the dosage without the advice of your physician. If you refill the prescription, you must not take again the initial, large digitalization dose but should simply continue the prescribed maintenance dose.

What Are the Symptoms of Digitalis Overdose?

They may include loss of appetite, nausea or vomiting, and weight loss. Usually, these are followed by headache, neuralgia, and malaise. Delirium and convulsions may occur with a large overdose; older people are particularly prone to becoming confused.

In very severe digitalis intoxication from overdose, the patient may see spots before the eyes, experience a flickering sensation, or see different colors.

Allergic skin rashes are rare. Men sometimes may have an enlargement of one or both breasts, but this is harmless.

Actually, the early symptoms—such as appetite loss, nausea, vomiting, and sometimes diarrhea—are undesirable but not serious. And they provide a convenient warning indication that the dose may be too high. If they occur, you should report them promptly to your physician so the dose may be properly adjusted.

It is possible that overdosage may cause heart rhythm disturbances. In such cases, an electrocardiogram may be necessary.

Usually, symptoms of intoxication can be dealt with adequately by eliminating or cutting down on the dosage temporarily, correcting any potassium deficiency, omitting diuretics for a time, and using medication to regulate heart rhythm. In rare instances a temporary pacemaker may be necessary.

After the symptoms are brought under control and blood

levels are corrected, the administration of digitalis can be resumed, usually at a lower dosage. It may also be advisable to omit taking the drug once or twice a week.

If you let your physician know promptly in the event that you experience any of the early symptoms just discussed, the likelihood of a serious reaction is remote—and if one should occur, it can be corrected.

Digitalis, as I've indicated and should emphasize again, is one of the oldest, most widely used and effective drugs for the heart. Don't be afraid of taking it if prescribed by your physician.

DIURETICS

What Exactly Are Diuretics?

Sometimes referred to as "water pills," diuretics are drugs that eliminate excess fluid from the body. They are often used for heart disease and hypertension.

By increasing urine excretion, and hence the removal of excess fluids, they lighten the load on the heart. And by increasing the salt excretion activity of the kidneys, diuretics can lower blood pressure.

Early diuretic agents included derivatives of caffeine. As you undoubtedly know, coffee and tea act as weak diuretics (because of their content of caffeine). Then came more modern diuretics—compounds of mercury such as mercaptomerin and meralluride, which proved most useful when given by injection.

In recent years has come a whole series of diuretics that are effective when taken by mouth. They include drugs of the thiazide family—among them, chlorothiazide, hydrochlorothiazide, trichlormethiazide, bendroflumethiazide, polythiazide, benzthiazide, and hydroflumethiazide. There are also diuretics of the phthalimidine family, which includes chlorthalidone. And there are others as well, such as spironolactone, theophylline, and ethacrynic acid.

Essentially, the different diuretics are similar in action, although sometimes one may be more effective than another for a particular patient. As they act on the kidneys to increase the removal by those organs of sodium (salt) and water from the blood and these are excreted in the urine, the sodium and water are replaced from the water-loaded tissues.

Diuretics are usually given in tablet form and some are effective within an hour or two and may remain active for twelve to twenty-four hours.

If necessary, when a patient has severe heart failure and elimination of fluid accumulation is urgent, a powerful diuretic given by injection may, within fifteen to twenty minutes, lead to a significant increase in urine flow and relief of shortness of breath caused by fluid congestion of the lungs.

Do Diuretics Have Any Side Effects?

They may in some patients.

There is a long list of possible side effects. Needless to say, they do not all occur together, nor is it probable that most of them will occur at all.

The possible side effects include skin rash, extreme weakness, dizziness, lethargy, drowsiness, low blood pressure, nausea, vomiting, muscle cramps, and extreme thirst and dry mouth, especially if kidney or liver function is impaired for other reasons.

As diuretics increase fluid excretion, they also increase excretion of certain salts. Thus, the risk of digitalis side effects increases if you take diuretics, since the effect of digitalis increases greatly with low body levels of potassium or magnesium salts. To prevent this, if you are taking digitalis and a diuretic, your physician may recommend that you drink unsweetened orange juice or eat a banana daily. Oranges and bananas are rich in potassium.

Your physician may recommend that you take potassium in the form of a special table salt. This should not be confused with ordinary table salt, which contains sodium. An excess intake of ordinary salt should be avoided if you are taking a diuretic. As an alternative, your physician may recommend that you take a potassium chloride solution.

If you are taking both a diuretic and digitalis, your physician will order periodic blood tests to check on the concentrations of such electrolytes, as they are called, as potassium. Deficiencies usually can be readily corrected if they occur.

Diuretics sometimes may tend to increase the level of uric acid in the blood, precipitating an attack of gout manifested by a swollen, tender big toe or other joint. Such an attack can be overcome by medication and future occurrences can be prevented. In some cases, a diuretic may increase blood-sugar levels and hence increase the requirements for insulin or for oral medication used to control diabetes.

There are other side effects that are even more rare—skin rash, small bruises of the skin, oversensitivity to sunlight, deficiencies in white blood cells or anemia due to red blood cell deficiencies. If they occur, such reactions can be treated. Usually, the physician will discontinue the drug causing the reactions and it is best not taken again.

Do not be alarmed by the many possible side effects. They are *possible,* but *rare.* The reason for listing them is to make you aware of them. With early detection, your physician can use measures to overcome them. If you believe that you are experiencing any one or more, by all means let your physician know at once. Sometimes the measures for overcoming side effects are very simple indeed.

The beneficial effects of diuretics far outweigh their possible side effects.

NITROGLYCERIN

What's the Purpose of Nitroglycerin?

Nitroglycerin, like digitalis, is another old drug with remarkable value. It's prescribed to overcome attacks of anginal chest pain, which it can commonly do with great speed. And it's also prescribed to reduce the frequency or even prevent many angina attacks.

It comes in several forms. The most common is a small tablet that is placed under the tongue when chest pain is felt or in anticipation of a situation that can be expected to cause such pain.

Don't swallow such a tablet. It will do little good if swallowed. It is most effective under the tongue where it is dissolved by saliva and rapidly absorbed, producing almost instantaneous relief.

There are long-acting forms of nitroglycerin and similar drugs, in tablet and capsule form. Some, such as isosorbide dinitrate (trade-named Sorbitrate and Isordil), are taken under the tongue like nitroglycerin. Some are chewed and some others are swallowed. Among other long-acting agents are nitroglycerin in a special form (trade-named Nitro-bid), erythrityl tetranitrate (Cardilate), pentaerithritol tetranitrate (Peritrate), and long-acting isosorbide tablets (Isordil Tembids).

The long-lasting agents take longer to act as well and so they are not useful in treating angina if it is already present but rather may be used to prevent chest pain.

Nitroglycerin also comes in the form of an ointment, the effects of which last for several hours. It should be applied to the chest or other parts of the body and is particularly helpful when angina wakes you during the night. When applied before going to sleep, nitroglycerin ointment may prevent such attacks.

Physicians do not quite know how nitroglycerin relieves anginal pain. You'll recall that angina is a kind of cry of the heart against being overburdened, against being asked to put out more effort than it can readily do because it isn't getting enough oxygen.

By expanding the coronary arteries that feed the heart muscle, nitroglycerin gets more oxygen to the heart. It also expands blood vessels in the rest of the body and in doing so decreases the amount of work the heart has to do in pumping blood.

Remember that angina does not mean that you are having a heart attack. Nitroglycerin will almost always help relieve pain caused by angina.

Needless to say, when taking nitroglycerin for an angina attack, you should also stop the activity that brought on the pain. Just be calm and sit still for a short time until the nitroglycerin works.

Are There Side Effects?

At times there may be a few. But measured against the great usefulness of the medication, these side effects are usually worth bearing and actually are minimal.

You may experience a pounding headache for a short time because the blood vessels in your brain as well as the coronary vessels are expanded. There may be a slight burning sensation under the tongue.

Neither of these two side effects should worry you. They show that the medication is working and they usually become milder after you have used the tablets for a time.

Sometimes a harmless flushing of the face may occur. At other times dizziness or faintness may be experienced especially while standing, caused by a blood-pressure drop and too rapid or too slow a pulse. For this reason, until you become used to the medication, take it while sitting or lying down. If faintness and dizziness still occur you should consult your physician.

How Long Is Nitroglycerin Good For? Does It Deteriorate?

An important point. Yes, it does deteriorate.

Always keep it in a dark bottle and don't keep it for more than six months. It should cause a slight burning sensation when placed under your tongue. If it doesn't, discard it and get a fresh supply. A newer form of the drug (Nitrostat) is claimed to last a full year.

When and How Often Should I Take It?

Your physician will instruct you to take nitroglycerin to relieve angina—which, of course, causes discomfort or pain in the chest, usually characterized by a feeling of tightness, squeezing or pressing feelings, burning sensations, sensations of heaviness, ballooning pressure, or any other chest discomfort. At times, the discomfort may be in the upper-mid abdomen.

You should also take nitroglycerin for cardiac pain in the throat, jaws, gums, lower teeth, shoulders, back (between the shoulder blades), arms, wrists, hands, and fingers. Such pain may occur during physical stress, cold weather, excitement, or after eating a meal. Occasionally, it may occur without such stress. Instead of pain in the arms the discomfort may be manifested by only a mild aching, numbness, weakness, or a tingling sensation.

You should not be stoic and tolerate the pain of angina. Don't hesitate to take nitroglycerin.

It is also advisable for you to take it before you do anything that you must do even though you have reason to believe it will trigger an angina attack.

Should you experience angina on leaving your home, after eating, upon walking to your car, while shopping, moving your bowels, during sexual intercourse, or during working, feel free to take a nitroglycerin tablet two to three minutes before these activities. It frequently will prevent the angina.

There may be many occasions when you need nitroglycerin. Therefore, always have it in your pocket, kept in a tightly closed dark bottle. The pocket should not be too close to your body.

How Many Nitroglycerin Tablets May I Take?

If the first tablet is not effective in relieving an attack of angina, you can take another in two or three minutes. And if this is not enough, take a third tablet, two or three minutes after the second. Feel free with your physician's approval to take three tablets in this manner if necessary, but do not take more than three for any one attack.

If the angina does not subside within fifteen minutes, call your physician. If you cannot reach him or her immediately, have yourself taken without delay to the nearest hospital emergency room. Remain calm, don't panic, but get there quickly.

Do not drive yourself. If necessary, call a mobile heart unit, ambulance, or fire department emergency unit.

If you have heart disease, you should plan ahead for the quickest way to get help if it ever should be needed. Such an emergency plan may help save your life if an emergency arises. Have the proper telephone numbers available for ready use. Discuss the plan with your family beforehand.

Don't become excited. It may be a false alarm, but if pain persists and recurs frequently it could mean that you are having a heart attack. It is better to play it safe and get to the hospital where the best care can be provided.

Don't panic because of the pain. Try nitroglycerin first. The chances of its working are excellent. If it doesn't work, however, get to help quickly.

Can I Use Nitroglycerin More Than Once During the Same Day?

Yes, you can—and should. Use it as often as pain recurs or when you are going into situations that you expect may provoke an angina attack.

If pain recurs many times during the day, however, it is important that you call your physician for advice. Frequently recurring angina—especially if that represents a dramatic change from your previous pattern of angina—should be treated in a hospital.

PROPRANOLOL (INDERAL)

What's the Nature and Purpose of This Drug?

Propranolol (trade-named Inderal) is a member of a relatively new class of drugs called beta blockers. It is used because it has a blocking action against certain substances that circulate in the bloodstream and can cause the heart to beat faster and stronger. It also decreases nerve impulses, which have the same effects on the heart.

Propranolol therefore acts to relax the heart somewhat and to make it beat more slowly and less forcefully. When the heart beats more slowly, it needs less oxygen. And a heart that needs less oxygen is less likely to cause angina, which is brought on by a shortage of oxygen.

In addition, propranolol has an action similar to that of quinidine (page 164). It smooths out certain disturbances in the heart's rhythm.

Propranolol is employed in some cases of high blood pressure. And it can also be used to decrease a rapid pulse rate in patients with an overactive thyroid gland.

For a heart disease patient, propranolol is usually prescribed for the relief of angina when nitroglycerin alone is no longer sufficient to overcome pain and discomfort. This should be accompanied by other measures such as changes in one's life-style, including the elimination of smoking and avoidance as much as possible of great stress and undue reactions to stress.

Propranolol comes in orange-colored 10-milligram tablets, green-colored 40-milligram tablets, and yellow-colored 80-milligram tablets. In case of an emergency, it can also be given by injection into a vein.

The optimal amount of the drug varies from person to person and with the severity of the disease. When the drug is taken the pulse rate usually decreases, but the dose should be adjusted so as not to allow it to go below 50 to 55 beats a minute.

Propranolol may sometimes be used in combination with a long-acting nitroglycerin preparation for combating angina. Long-acting nitroglycerin can be taken after meals and at bedtime. Propranolol may be taken several times a day. Both, if necessary, may be taken more often and at night when prescribed by your physician. The peak action of these drugs lasts only a few hours.

Propranolol is often used in combination with still other drugs. The precise combination of drugs best for your heart is a matter of the most delicate medical decision. And it is important that you inform your physician immediately about any effects and side-effects of prescribed medications so he or she can arrive at the optimal both in terms of combination and in terms of dosage.

It's very important to note this about propranolol: Its use must not be discontinued abruptly, otherwise the heart's need for oxygen may rise suddenly and this may possibly bring on a heart attack.

If propranolol is to be discontinued for any reason, its use should be slowly decreased over a period of several days to two weeks.

If you are going to have surgery of any kind, be sure that the surgeon knows you are using propranolol. Its presence in the body can complicate the effects of anesthesia. Some physicians discontinue the drug gradually and omit it completely for two days prior to surgery.

Does Propranolol Have Any Side Effects?

Under certain conditions, the drug can be lifesaving. But like many drugs, it may have side effects.

During the hay fever season, if you have that problem, it may increase your allergic reaction. If you have a history of asthma, the drug may make the asthma worse or precipitate allergic attacks.

Sometimes propranolol may slow your heart and/or lower your blood pressure too much. Therefore, both you and a member of your family should learn how to take your pulse.

The pulse is usually taken just below the base of the thumb, on the inside of the wrist. Place the tips of two or three fingers over this point and apply light pressure in order to feel the pulse. Don't use your thumb, since it has a pulse of its own that can be confusing. Count the pulse for one minute using a timepiece with a second hand.

If your pulse at rest falls below a rate of 50 beats a minute, you should report that to your physician. On the other hand, should you still experience frequent angina attacks and your pulse rate remains over 50 beats a minute, you should report that to your physician as well. The dosage of propranolol may be increased.

You should also call your physician if you become short-winded or cough a lot at night, and if this interferes with sleep. It may be the result of inability of your heart to pump enough blood, a weakness occasionally caused by propranolol. In that case, your physician may readjust the dosage or add other drugs such as digitalis or a diuretic. This will usually improve your condition. If it does not, your physician may further adjust or discontinue the propranolol.

There are other side effects associated with propranolol that occur much less frequently. They include numbness of the hands, light-headedness, weakness, sleeping difficulty, depression, forgetfulness, confusion, nausea, vomiting, abdominal cramps, diarrhea, constipation, rash, fever, hair loss, and blue spots on the skin. These reactions are usually reversible with a change of dosage or elimination of the drug.

As with any medication, your physician will prescribe propranolol only if he or she believes that the benefits outweigh any risks. So if your physician has prescribed it you should not be afraid of it. The good it does will probably far outweigh any possible harm from side effects—particularly if you consult with your physician immediately upon noticing any of the reactions I've indicated and remain under his or her close supervision at all times.

QUINIDINE

What's the Value of Quinidine?

This drug, which is derived from the bark of the tropical cinchona tree and is related to quinine, is an effective anti-arrhythmic agent.

Its principal effect is the elimination or reduction of excessive impulses within the heart that can lead to premature beats and episodes of rapid heart action.

It is usually given in tablet form but occasionally may be injected into a muscle. And in addition to stopping abnormal heart rhythms, it can be used to help prevent recurrences.

A simple blood test can be used to monitor the level of quinidine in the blood so the dosage can be adjusted to need.

What Are the Side Effects?

Side effects can occur, usually when the dose is too high.

These reactions may include ear noises, impairment of hearing, dizziness, double vision, spots before the eyes, reduction in the size of the visual field, diarrhea, or fever.

Sometimes quinidine may cause, rather than correct, disturbances in the heart rhythm. Occasionally, a patient may be unusually sensitive to the drug, even to a small dose. Usually such sensitivity becomes obvious in the first few weeks of use, with the appearance of small red or bluish spots on the skin, of bleeding from the nose, or of blood in the stool or in the urine. This reaction may be due to a decrease in the level in the blood of platelets, which are tiny disk-shaped bodies that initiate blood clotting.

If you should notice any of these signs, stop taking the quinidine at once and contact your physician immediately. Tell him or her what you have noticed and that you have stopped taking the drug. Ask for further advice.

If your physician thinks you need quinidine, you are very likely to benefit from it. And more than likely your physician can hold side effects to a minimum. You should have a regular blood platelet count. This is a simple blood test and usually provides a reliable warning signal about one of the possibly serious side effects of quinidine.

PROCAINAMIDE
(Pronestyl®)

What Does Procainamide Do?

Procainamide—a drug originally used as a local anesthetic and related to the well-known Novocain—is an anti-arrhythmic drug.

It is similar in action to quinidine but is shorter lasting. One drug or the other may be preferable for some patients.

In an emergency situation, when it is necessary to overcome rapid heart action quickly, procainamide has an advantage over quinidine in that it is safer when injected into a vein, which is a route of administration that gets a drug into the system quickly.

For oral use procainamide comes in 250-milligram, 375-milligram, and 500-milligram capsules and tablets. Because it has a shorter action than quinidine in some patients it may have to be taken every three to four hours around the clock to assure smooth, continuous action.

In order to insure that you are getting the correct dosage, it is best to keep a total daily dose of procainamide—and any other drug you are taking for your heart—in a container that you can keep accessible during the day, since often the business of the day makes one forget whether or not medication has been taken.

What Are the Side Effects?

Side effects may sometimes occur either because of a dosage too high for your body or because of unusual sensitivity to the drug. They are more likely in the presence of heart failure or kidney failure.

The side effects can include loss of appetite, nausea, hives, itching, reduced blood pressure. Procainamide can also cause sore throat or upper respiratory infection accompanied by fever. It may lower the count of white cells in your blood; these cells, also known as leukocytes, are part of the body's defense system against infection.

After several months of use, procainamide may sometimes cause rash, fever, joint aches and swellings, chest pain on breathing, and fluid accumulation in the chest. This syndrome, or complex of symptoms, is called drug-induced lupus.

Sometimes procainamide, like quinidine, may cause heart rhythm disturbances.

If a new rhythm disturbance or any other side effect occurs, immediately discontinue the drug and notify your physician so he can alleviate the side effect, prevent progression of possibly dangerous complications, and replace procainamide with another drug when indicated.

Although side effects from procainamide can become serious, serious complications can be minimized or prevented if you watch for the symptoms I've mentioned, stop taking the drug should any occur, and contact your physician.

Your doctor will be able to confirm any toxic effect by specific blood tests—such as a white cell count, lupus cell preparation, or anti-nuclear factor determination.

Usually, if reactions do occur and the drug is stopped they gradually disappear without any specific treatment. In rare cases, procainamide can be continued and another drug added to overcome the side effects.

Disopyramide (Norpace), a new, recently released anti-arrhythmic drug, may sometimes be effective in cases where other anti-arrhythmic drugs have failed or are not tolerated by the patient.

ANTICOAGULANTS: COUMADIN®–DICUMAROL–HEPARIN

What Purpose Do Anticoagulants Serve?

Coagulation is the changing of a liquid into a thickened or solid material. When that happens in the blood, a clot is formed.

Anticoagulants are compounds that overcome a tendency to clotting within the heart and blood vessels. And they may be used in heart patients when it is considered necessary to overcome such a tendency.

There are two basic kinds of anticoagulants. One is represented by heparin, which works directly on the clotting mechanism of blood. It interferes with the series of chemical events that must take place in blood in order for clotting to occur.

The other type, represented by Coumadin and Dicumarol,

acts in another way. These compounds work in the liver. The liver produces prothrombin, which is a factor present in the blood and required for clotting. Coumadin and Dicumarol interfere with the liver's formation of prothrombin.

The choice of an anticoagulant will depend upon a particular patient's need.

Coumadin and Dicumarol are usually given by mouth. One or the other may be used just once a day.

Heparin is given by injection, either directly into a vein every four hours or as a continuous infusion or sometimes just under the skin every eight to twelve hours. Should your physician determine that you need heparin over the long term, you will be taught how to inject it, much as diabetic patients are taught to administer their own insulin.

Coumadin and Dicumarol should be avoided during pregnancy or when pregnancy is supected, because it may cause bleeding or malformation of the fetus. Heparin, on the other hand, can be given to pregnant women and to women who are nursing babies.

Why Are Blood Tests Needed When Anticoagulants Are Taken?

When an anticoagulant is used, its effects must be carefully evaluated if clotting is to be prevented without at the same time risking internal bleeding or profuse bleeding from even a minor cut. With blood tests, your physician can monitor the effects and determine the exact dosage you need.

When heparin is used, a test can measure clotting time in a sample of your blood. When Coumadin or Dicumarol is used, the blood test checks the prothrombin level to see that it is not reduced so much as to allow hemorrhaging.

At the beginning, before the exact dosage you need may be known, blood testing will be more frequent. Later the intervals between tests may be lengthened and your physician may request a test only every few weeks.

Do not think that you are getting worse if you should need a larger dosage of anticoagulant, or getting better if you should need less. The clotting time of blood may vary for reasons that we don't quite understand.

What Side Effects May Occur?

There may be signs and symptoms associated with a tendency to bleed easily.

You may find that you develop black-and-blue spots without having been bruised—because of some bleeding into the skin. You may also have nosebleeds—and you may find blood in the urine because of bleeding in the urinary tract or red or black blood in the stools because of bleeding in the stomach or intestines. In women, bleeding may occur from the vagina. Bleeding into the brain may cause headaches. Bleeding into the abdomen may cause severe abdominal pain.

If you experience such symptoms, stop the medication immediately and call your physician. He or she may use vitamin K to neutralize the action of an oral anticoagulant, if that is what you are using, and that will stop the bleeding. A drug called protamine sulphate can be used to neutralize heparin.

Sometimes bleeding may occur despite satisfactory blood tests, suggesting that there may be a cause other than use of an anticoagulant. In that case, your physician will carry out examinations and tests to uncover the hidden cause.

There are a few other possible side effects, less severe than bleeding. They include skin rash, nausea, cramps, diarrhea, and fever. If these occur, contact your physician immediately and follow the advice given.

Is It Safe to Take Other Drugs When an Anticoagulant Is Used?

This is an important question. Sometimes other medications, when used along with an anticoagulant, can increase the risk of bleeding. That's true of all aspirin-containing products. And, in addition to plain aspirin itself, there are many such products.

You should know that the following contain aspirin: Norgesic, Darvon Compound, Phenaphen, Fiorinal, Percodan, Robaxisal, Zactirin, Daprisal, Ecotrin, some Alka-Seltzer preparations, Coricidin, Coricidin "D", Dristan, Novahistine with A.P.C., Super-Anahist, Triaminicin, Anacin, A.P.C., A.S.A. Compound, Ascriptin, Aspergum, Bufferin, Cama Inlay-Tabs, Capron Capsules, Cope, Counterpain, Derfort, Derfule, Dolor, Empirin Compound, Excedrin, Liquiprin, Measurin, Midol, P-A-C Compound, Phensal, Sal-Fayne, Stanback, Trigesic, and Vanquish.

Whereas aspirin and aspirin-containing products—and alcohol as well—may lead to bleeding when you take an anticoagulant, some drugs, such as phenobarbitol and other sedatives, may interfere with anticoagulant action.

You should be very careful about taking drugs you can get without prescription. And you should be careful, too, about prescription medications—informing any new physician who may treat you for your heart or for any other problem that you are taking an anticoagulant. It's important that you do not receive deep injections into a muscle while taking an anticoagulant, since that may lead to bleeding into the muscle.

Must I Receive an Anticoagulant If I Have a Heart Attack?

About a decade or so ago, anticoagulants were administered routinely to heart attack patients. This was done to prevent further blood-clot formation and to help dissolve existing clots.

Today, however, physicians are uncertain about the need for and value of such treatment, and anticoagulants are not always prescribed as a matter of course.

It is now recognized that while a heart attack may be caused by a clot in a coronary artery or branch, it may also occur without such a clot. Blood clots are not found in a substantial number of patients in the early stages of a heart attack. And it appears that a heart attack can occur when, in the absence of a clot, a severe spasm or sudden narrowing of an artery or branch occurs.

Moreover, the evidence for the value of anticoagulants after heart attacks is not clear-cut. Some studies indicate that the drugs are beneficial; some, that they provide no particular benefit; others, that they may cause harm.

Today, most physicians prescribe anticoagulants only under specific circumstances. They may do so if a patient has a history of blood clots in the veins (thrombophlebitis) or in the lungs before the heart attack or if the patient shows signs of an excessive tendency toward clotting during recovery from the attack.

Anticoagulants may also be used in cases of extreme obesity, if the heart does not pump adequate amounts of blood, if the patient is young, or if there has been a previous heart attack causing clots within the heart chambers.

On the other hand, anticoagulants are usually avoided under such conditions as severe high blood pressure, kidney failure, or active stomach ulcers, or if there is to be surgery on the brain, spinal cord, prostate, or other internal organ. (In fact, if you have been placed on an anticoagulant and the occasion arises when you need any kind of surgery, even including tooth extraction, you should let the surgeon or dentist know that you are on an anticoagulant.)

Whether or not you will receive an anticoagulant may well depend upon your physician's conviction as to its possible value. Some physicians who prescribe anticoagulants do so in the hope of dissolving a blood clot. Others who do not prescribe them rely on the heart's ability to heal itself, the formation of a firm scar, and the formation of new blood vessels that may grow through a thrombus and make blood flow possible again.

Because evidence in favor of one or the other approach is not yet conclusive, either is sensible in the light of present knowledge.

I expect that, along with many others, you may find this a bit confusing. Yet differences in methods of treatment not only for heart problems but for many other conditions are often inevitable because of the complexity of medicine.

If, you may ask, there is conflicting evidence about the value of anticoagulants after a heart attack, why should any physician use them? Yet, were physicians always to wait for conclusive scientific proof before attempting any reasonably safe method of treatment, many patients would suffer unnecessarily. Treatment may be decided not only on the basis of scientific proof but also on the basis of clinical experience.

Whether you receive anticoagulant treatment or not may, then, be determined by your physician's experience over many years in treating patients such as yourself. You will be treated according to what your physician's training and experience indicate may be best for you.

Despite the complexities of medicine, it is a gratifying fact that much progress has been made—that, for example, your chance of leaving the hospital alive and improved after a heart attack are about twice as great as they would have been ten years ago.

Don't try to compare every last detail of your treatment with that of others. Once you have a physician, leave the judgments and decisions—and worries—to him or her. On the other hand, you have every right to inquire whether your physician is competent and has kept up with modern medical practice. And if you have any doubts on this score, don't be afraid to ask for a consultation with another physician. No conscientious physician should object to such a request and he or she should guide you in choosing an experienced consultant.

ASPIRIN AND VITAMIN E

Can Aspirin Prevent Heart Disease?

Aspirin decreases the activity of blood platelets which, as we have noted earlier, are involved in blood clotting.

Some physicians, hoping to decrease heart attacks and strokes, may prescribe aspirin. As yet, scientific studies have not confirmed that aspirin has any significant beneficial effects on the occurrence or recurrence of heart attacks. Studies are continuing.

Aspirin should not, as we have noted, be taken with anticoagulants since it may then cause bleeding.

Nor should you, under any circumstances, try to treat

yourself with aspirin, hoping to prevent or overcome a heart attack. Heart disease is complex. It requires expert treatment.

Can Vitamin E Help?

Ever since 1935 when it was isolated from wheat-germ oil, vitamin E has been controversial because of claims that have made it seem to be a panacea for most ills.

At various times and by various people, including some physicians, vitamin E has been hailed as a means of increasing male potency and assuring orgasm in women; of improving sperm quality and chances of conception; of preventing miscarriage and reducing the likelihood of birth deformities. Beyond all that, it has also been reputed to be a way of treating and preventing high blood pressure, gangrene, the kidney disease nephritis, varicose veins, and atherosclerosis and heart attacks.

Yet there is no established scientific proof for any of this—and certainly not for heart disease.

Vitamin E is found in abundance in whole grains but is almost nonexistent in refined white flour. Other foods rich in it include fresh beef liver, wheat germ, fruits and green leafy vegetables, margarine, mayonnaise, nuts, and vegetable oils, including corn, peanut, and soya oils.

According to some studies, the daily requirement of vitamin E in adults is 30 I.U. (International Units) in men and 25 in women. That amount should be readily obtainable in a good balanced and varied diet. An increased intake of polyunsaturated fats increases vitamin E requirements.

Vitamin E deficiency is rare in adults. A deficiency can cause anemia. It does so in some infants, especially those fed formulas high in unsaturated oils. The infants respond to vitamin E supplementation. In adults, red blood cell life may be abnormally shortened by a deficiency of vitamin E.

Overdosage of vitamin E appears to be harmless, although some investigators have reported that large doses may cause cholesterol to be deposited in the inner lining of the aorta in rats and may be associated with increased growth of lung tumors in mice.

While there have been no conclusive scientific studies showing that large doses of the vitamin are beneficial to the heart and blood vessel system, a few physicians recommend vitamin E—based on clinical impressions—in such conditions as angina, heart attacks, and blood vessel pain in the legs.

They have the impression that angina may be improved and the danger of heart attack decreased. They also have the impression that the vitamin may avoid atherosclerosis in leg arteries and blood clotting in veins and in the lungs. They indicate that vitamin E may do this by decreasing the need for oxygen, decreasing the tendency for blood to clot, and dilating blood vessels in the extremities.

Since there is no scientific proof of vitamin E's effectiveness, nor good reason to think it harmful, you can probably do what you wish about using it. Have no illusions, however, that the vitamin can, in any way, replace heart medication, medical supervision, carefully controlled diet, and elimination of risk factors.

PACEMAKERS

Of What Use Are Pacemakers?

Electronic pacemakers now are keeping the hearts of thousands of people beating well and regularly despite chronic heart disease.

The heart has its own natural pacemaker and an electrical conduction system that control its rhythm and coordinate its contractions. As mentioned earlier (Chapter 2), the natural pacemaker is a small area of specialized tissue located in the upper right part of the heart. A group of cells in this tissue sends out electrical impulses, which travel along conduction pathways and stimulate the heart muscle to contract rhythmically.

The whole system, of course, depends on the coronary ar-

Heart Medications and Heart Pacemakers

teries to bring adequate oxygen and nutrition for the heart. If there should be a blockage of a coronary artery or branch, as in a heart attack, proper functioning of the system may be disturbed. The heart may beat irregularly or too slowly.

Usually, medication can overcome such disturbances. Occasionally, however, it may fail to do so. In such cases, an electronic pacemaker can be used. A pacemaker can restore the proper heartbeat and, in doing so, can be lifesaving.

How Does a Pacemaker Work?

Much as does the heart's natural pacemaker.

The electronic device starts the contraction or pumping action of the heart by sending a tiny electrical signal into the heart muscle by means of a small insulated wire called an electrode. The electrode is either attached from the outside of the heart directly to the muscle or threaded through a vein and lodged inside the heart. The tip of the electrode is actually a conductive metal through which the electrical charge is delivered to the muscle. The strength of that charge is so slight that it usually cannot be felt.

A pacemaker may be needed only temporarily. In that case, an external device is used. The pacemaker itself remains outside the body, and wires from it are moved up, in a simple procedure under a local anesthetic, through a vein, into the right auricle and/or ventricle of the heart.

When the pacemaker is then turned on, it substitutes for the natural pacemaker and maintains a regular heart action. When the heart rhythm becomes normal again on its own, the electronic pacemaker is no longer needed and the wires can be almost painlessly removed. This may happen in a matter of a few days or a week or two.

What If the Pacemaker Is Needed Permanently?

That's necessary when the heart system is damaged beyond the point of healing. Then a permanent pacemaker, about the size of a pocket watch, can be inserted under the skin under local anesthesia. The entire procedure takes about an hour or less.

The first pacemakers were "fixed rate." That is, they gave off a continuous signal at a pre-set rate selected for the patient by his or her physician.

Later pacemakers—and these are now much more commonly used—are of the "demand" type. They have a special sensing circuit that monitors the normal electrical activity of the heart. As long as the heart rate—the number of beats per minute—remains above a prescribed level, the demand pacemaker remains inactive. If the patient's heart rate drops below that level, however, the demand unit immediately begins sending impulses to regulate the beat.

Can I Live a Normal Life With a Pacemaker?

Yes, you can. You may play golf, swim, dance—in short, engage in all activities you enjoyed before there was any trouble with your natural pacemaker and conduction system.

However, a few precautions are necessary when you have a pacemaker. For instance, you must avoid certain microwave stoves and electric shavers. And you must stay away from strong magnets. These devices can affect the operation of the pacemaker.

You will usually be taught to count your own pulse rate. If it should drop more than five beats a minute below your normal rate, a change of batteries may be needed. Or, since batteries usually last five years or more, it may be necessary only to adjust the wires.

If at any time you experience faintness, dizziness, or rapid heart action, you should either immediately contact your physician or go to a hospital emergency room for an adjustment of the pacemaker.

Pacemakers are generally reliable and remarkably effective.

8

Heart Surgery

Coronary bypass surgery—sometimes also called coronary revascularization—is a procedure designed to bring more blood to the heart muscle, detouring it around blocked portions of the coronary arteries. When might it be useful, its benefits outweighing risks? What's involved? When it's successful, how successful is it? In this chapter I answer these and other questions about a procedure that has been much publicized, does have value for some heart patients, but has its limitations and may or may not be advisable for you. And I indicate when your physician may wish you to consider it for yourself.

Under What Conditions Should Bypass Surgery Be Considered?

When you suffer from intolerable anginal pain, with very frequent and severe attacks, with poor response to adequate medical care.

I emphasize "adequate." Such care should include thorough efforts to find medical treatment that might be helpful, perhaps involving trials of a number of medications and combinations of medications. And not medication alone, but also possible changes in life-style, such as temporary rest, appropriate diet, elimination of smoking.

When such a program carried out for a reasonable length

of time, supervised by a cardiologist, has been tried and has failed, then you should be asked to consider bypass surgery. It should also be considered if your physician tells you that your main anterior coronary artery is badly clogged, for clogging of this particular artery, when severe, can represent a major threat of massive heart attack.

In all other circumstances, there is no clear-cut answer as to who lives longer, the medically or surgically treated patient. This uncertainty created the need for a large ongoing collaborative study supported by the National Institutes of Health. The study, at thirteen medical centers, will try to find out whether coronary bypass surgery does or does not prolong life for patients with angina or for patients who have recovered from a heart attack.

In considering surgery, you should be fully aware of its limitations.

What Are the Limitations?

It would be nice if surgery could cure coronary artery disease. But it doesn't. It can't. The underlying disease process—which leads to the development of clogging deposits in the arteries—is not something surgery can do anything for or about.

Any hope of preventing that atherosclerotic process—or of retarding or preventing its further progression—lies in attention to the risk factors discussed earlier. I'm sure you will understand that basic fact.

Although it is not curative, bypass surgery can still provide relief in a large proportion of cases when it is clearly indicated for very severe and otherwise unyielding angina and for main anterior coronary artery obstruction.

But that relief may or may not be lasting. There can be no absolute guarantee that it will be. Why? First because if the underlying atherosclerotic process continues to advance, it may produce clogging of another coronary artery or branch or even clogging at some point in a bypassed artery beyond the bypass. And, second, because there is always some risk that the bypass itself may become choked and occluded or lose its patency or openness.

The cost of the operation, too, needs consideration as you weigh its potential benefits and risks.

May Cost Be a Major Consideration?

The cost is extraordinarily high, especially should prolonged hospitalization be required because of complications.

If you are not wealthy, you should, before agreeing to have surgery, obtain from your surgeon a fairly precise estimate of all the costs you may incur, including those that may arise should any complications develop. And you should then determine the resources you have, including the exact extent of coverage by your insurance, for payment of all the expenses.

It may not seem to be a proper medical concern to advise you to consider finances in the light of your medical condition and possible need. But should the high costs lead to financial distress for you and your family, your worry and anxiety about that will not be helpful.

You should have an idea—after thorough discussion with your cardiologist and with the surgeon—about the possibility of complications, about how long you will need to be hospitalized after the operation, and how long before you can return to gainful work.

Does the Operation Prolong Life?

We just do not know as yet. There is no proof that it will or will not—except possibly in the relatively few cases of a severely diseased main anterior coronary artery when it may well add years to life.

The bypass procedure is being performed with increasing frequency throughout the country. There has been much publicity about it.

You should be aware that it has come into widespread use only in the last half-dozen years or so. As with any other new surgical procedure—and, for that matter, any new medical measure—it will take many more years of experience with it, of follow-up of long-term results in those who have undergone it, before there can be definitive information about the long-term results.

As of now, bypass surgery is considered to be still "on trial" and the opinion of experts about its value in prolonging life is divided.

It may well turn out to be life-prolonging. On the other hand, it may be judged in the long run not to have such value. That has been the case with several surgical procedures previously performed for the same purpose in the past, often with great enthusiasm. In the long run they proved to have no life-prolonging value and have since been given up entirely.

How Do I Decide Whether to Have the Operation or Not?

You can make your decision wisely after obtaining and considering all the facts and perhaps considering several medical opinions. You should, of course, know something about the operation itself and its background—and I will shortly give you information on that score.

I would suggest that you be particularly wary of bypass surgery if you are free of or almost free of disabling symptoms—if your angina is well controlled by medical measures. You will want to remember in that case that there is no proof that the operation will prolong your life or prevent heart attacks. And you will want to remember too that in any kind of major surgery there is always some risk. Certainly there is risk in bypass surgery, and we'll discuss that shortly.

I would suggest, too, that you be skeptical of the advice of any honest but overenthusiastic surgeon who may assure you of success and prolongation of life if you should undergo bypass surgery and warn you of doom and short life if you should refuse surgery. Seek help in making your decision by obtaining other medical opinions.

Heart Surgery

Tell Me About the Operation Itself. How Is It Done?

The operation, as it is performed today, has been built on the basis of many past efforts. One of the earliest of the modern surgical efforts to try to overcome advanced coronary artery disease goes back only to 1929. At that time, Dr. Claude Beck, a distinguished surgeon, tried irritating the heart with talc and scraping procedures. He hoped, by the irritation, to stimulate the formation of new blood channels. But the amount of increased blood flow, if any, could not be determined.

Then, near the end of World War II, Dr. Arthur Vineberg of the Royal Victoria Hospital in Montreal conceived the idea of bringing new blood supply to the ailing heart by making use of the internal mammary artery. This is an artery that runs down behind the chest wall, supplying blood to certain chest areas. Because other arteries also supply these areas, the internal mammary could be spared.

Dr. Vineberg's idea was to free the artery from its attachments to the chest wall, bring it over to the heart muscle, and place it in a little tunnel made in the heart muscle. His hope was that when the internal mammary was thus implanted it might give rise to small collateral blood vessels that would become hooked up to unblocked branch coronary vessels, thus providing blood for the heart through a new network.

Over the course of many years, first in experimental animals and then in severely afflicted human patients, Dr. Vineberg was able to show that this sometimes does happen. It may take as long as six months, however, before the new network is established and the patient begins to benefit.

Other surgeons began to seek ways to more immediately help patients who might not survive that long. They developed one technique in which they opened a blocked portion of a coronary artery and reamed out the clogging material. In another technique, they slit an artery, left the clogging material in place, and grafted on a patch of vein to enlarge the vessel.

But both of these procedures had quite limited use—in the relatively few patients with obstruction limited to only a short length of artery.

Then in the late 1960s came the saphenous vein graft technique, which is widely used today.

The saphenous vein is a large vein which runs the length of each leg, returning some of the blood from the leg to the heart. The saphenous vein can be spared since other veins can take over its work. And, in fact, this is the vein that is often removed in varicose vein surgery.

The vein is removed from a leg and carefully tested to make certain it is in good condition. A suitable length of it is then used. One end is attached to the aorta, the major trunkline artery emerging from the heart and carrying fresh blood. The other end is attached beyond the point of obstruction in a coronary artery.

Thus, fresh blood from the aorta is carried around the obstruction and is then transported by the remaining unobstructed part of the coronary artery to nourish the heart muscle.

When more than one coronary artery or coronary artery branch is obstructed, several such bypasses can be made.

Another bypassing method that may be used employs the internal mammary artery. Instead of placing one end of the artery in a tunnel in the heart muscle, however, many surgeons now attach it, in the same fashion as a saphenous vein, to a diseased coronary vessel beyond the point of obstruction. For some patients, both the saphenous vein and the internal mammary artery are used.

What Are the Steps in the Operation?

Typically, before surgery—before even a patient is considered to be a candidate for the operation—catheterization with X-ray movies is done, as described in Chapter 6.

As you'll recall, the movies reveal where an obstruction in a coronary vessel is located. They enable the surgeon to plan for the operation ahead of time.

In the operating room, the surgeon is assisted by a sizable team that may include assisting surgeons, anesthesiologists, nurses, a heart-lung machine technician, and a technician for the electronic equipment that monitors the patient throughout the operation.

The operation begins, once the patient is anesthetized, with an incision in a leg to remove a length of saphenous vein. At the same time, the patient's chest is opened.

When the vein has been tested and prepared and is ready, the patient is connected to the heart-lung machine. The machine takes over temporarily the work of both heart and lungs. It removes carbon dioxide from the blood, adds oxygen, and pumps the blood through the body.

The heart then may be stopped as two electrodes are briefly touched to it. This gives the surgeon a quieter field in which to work.

The bypass is then carried out, with the vein attached with suture or stitching material as fine as a human hair. If necessary, several bypasses are carried out in the same way.

When the bypassing is completed, the patient is disconnected from the heart-lung machine. It is possible then to get a measure, through instrumentation, of the improved blood flow to the heart muscle going through the bypasses.

When, at last, the patient's chest is closed and he or she is ready to go from operating room to recovery room, the total procedure may have taken 3 to 6 hours or even more.

After surgery, the patient spends several days in the intensive care unit where continuous monitoring is used to make certain that there are no complications—and, if complications should occur, that they can be dealt with immediately.

As with any other major operation, length of hospital stay can vary considerably. In some cases, it may be as short as ten days, possibly less, and some patients may be back at work in as little as four to six weeks.

What Are the Risks of Bypass Surgery?

This is a serious operation. The risk of death varies from less than 2 percent to more than 20 percent, depending upon the skill and experience of the surgeon and the individual patient's condition.

During or immediately after the operation, some 10 to 15 percent of patients experience a heart attack despite expert medical attention. A heart attack is dangerous wherever or whenever it occurs, although it is not necessarily fatal.

In a small proportion of patients, lung, kidney, brain, or liver complication may occur. There is also the possibility of infection.

Beyond the immediate risks, while surgery is most often successful, it is not always so. The vein or artery used for the bypass may occlude, or close up. This occurs in some 15 to 20 percent of patients. It usually causes a return of anginal pain, which sometimes may be worse than before surgery.

Is There Any Study That Indicates How Well Surgically Treated Patients Do in Comparison with the Medically Treated?

A recently reported study by the National Heart, Lung and Blood Institute did concern itself with comparisons. It found that many patients with severe angina responded well to medication and had fewer heart attacks after therapy than those who underwent bypass surgery. It concluded that the death rate was low and about equal for both treatments, that heart attacks occurred more often after surgery, and that anginal pain persisted more after medical treatment than after surgery.

In the four-year study, sponsored by the institute, doctors at eight medical centers across the country tested 288 patients. Of these, 147 received intensive drug therapy and 141 underwent bypass surgery.

Mortality in the six months after treatment was undertaken was 4.1 percent for the medical group and 5 percent for the surgical patients, not statistically different. In follow-up studies averaging twenty-four months, medical group mortality was 5 percent against 5.2 percent among surgical patients, again not statistically different.

In the period of study, 18 percent of the bypass patients suffered heart attacks against 10 percent of the medically treated group. In follow-up studies, the heart attack rate was equal for both groups.

The investigating physicians found that eventually one third of the medically treated patients required bypass surgery because of persistent pain. But the study indicated that delaying surgical treatment had no effect on mortality and that meant that two thirds of the medically treated group could be spared surgery. Thus, neither medical nor surgical treatment was proved superior except for one third of angina patients whose pain could not be controlled by drugs. Even in these patients, the mortality rate was not affected. Hopefully, an ongoing, larger study will remove remaining uncertainties.

If I Should Need Surgery, How Do I Choose a Surgeon?

Get your cardiologist's recommendation for the best surgeon for your operation. You may also wish to consult a second cardiologist—both to confirm the need for surgery and to get another recommendation for choice of a surgeon.

It is important to keep in mind that a surgeon usually becomes more skillful after doing many bypass procedures—at least one hundred of them. Moreover, to maintain his skill, he should do at least three such operations a week and should have the support of a competent, well-trained cardiac team.

It is entirely appropriate—indeed, advisable—for you to inquire about the mortality rate of the surgeon you are considering. Ask this question in the presence of a member of your family or a friend in order to avoid any misunderstanding.

The surgeon's mortality rate should compare favorably with the rate achieved in the major heart surgery centers, where it is reported to be less than 2 percent. Make certain that the mortality rate your surgeon quotes is *his or her own* and not that of the leading heart surgeons.

And it would be well for you to make similar inquiries

when it comes to the choice of the physician who will do the heart catheterization prior to surgery.

Does Surgery Ever Cure Heart Disease?

Yes—but these are the relatively rare forms of heart disease.

When it comes to various congenital heart defects—the defects that children are born with—surgeons today can accomplish remarkable feats. And very often they are curative.

In these congenital conditions, there may be a hole in the septum, or wall within the heart, that can be closed; a valve within the heart that does not work properly and can be repaired or, if necessary, replaced; or another defect that can be remedied.

But surgery cannot cure the most common form of heart disease—coronary heart disease.

Whether or Not I Have Surgery, Then, Will I Still Need to Pay Attention to Risk Factors and Life-Style?

Although medical treatment can provide some relief of symptoms, even possibly complete relief, surgical treatment may sometimes be needed for such relief. But if the course of the underlying atherosclerotic disease—which has given you concern and has made necessary medical or surgical treatment—is to be kept from progressing rapidly, it's essential that any and all risk factors that apply in your case be removed.

Some of those factors—such as excess weight, smoking, sedentary life-style, personality characteristics that exacerbate or even impose severe stress—are not easily overcome. Overcoming them may require a considerable, highly motivated effort. But you very probably have the motivation now and are capable of the effort.

And, of course, other risk factors—such as high blood pressure, diabetes, and gout—can be controlled by your physician with your cooperation.

9

Other Questions That Concern You and Your Family

How Should I React to a Member of My Family Who Has Had a Heart Attack?

You will naturally be concerned about someone you love. However, you should remember who is sick. While your loved one is in the hospital, do not let your fears and concerns show. The patient deserves all the encouragement you and the rest of the family can give.

At first, during the early acute stages of the attack, the patient usually will be heavily sedated since rest at this stage is very important. As the days pass, the patient will be less sedated and you will be able to be together more.

Do not bring up unpleasant or painful things such as unpaid bills, problems in your own life or anybody else's, bad news, or any problem in general. Don't burden the patient with complaints or even observations about any enforced changes in your life. Again, remember who is the patient—and that you are an important part of his or her recovery.

It's quite likely that the patient has many fears and worries about the family. Provide reassurance that you are all right and also that you are looking forward to doing things together again when he or she is well enough after leaving the hospital.

Is There Anything Else I Can Do?

It's likely that the patient is concerned about work and being able to resume it. The fact is that most patients with uncomplicated heart attacks are able to resume work. Most survive and become active again.

You may want to mention the experiences of Presidents Eisenhower and Johnson, pointing out that they both led active lives after their heart attacks. If you have mutual friends who have had similar experiences, you might cite them in your conversations, and you may want to invite them to pay the patient a visit.

A visit by the patient's boss often reduces the anxiety of the patient, especially if the boss shows genuine concern and reassures the patient that everybody at work misses him or her and that the job will be kept open—an assurance that will relieve financial worries.

The patient may also be worried about his or her sexual capacity. This, like all worries—if they are brought up by the patient—should be discussed by you with optimism and a complete willingness to wait until the time is right.

It is certainly not at all unusual for a patient to be depressed and worried after a heart attack. A major trauma has been experienced and a certain amount of sadness and anxiety is natural. You must provide support, assuring the patient that these are natural feelings and that the doubts will work themselves out in time.

By all means, encourage friends and your clergyman to visit. Don't smother the patient with sympathy. Though sick, he or she is an adult. Don't prevent the patient from carrying out the physician's instructions.

Be bright, cheerful, and optimistic—even if you don't feel that way. You have to put on a show, not only for the patient but for yourself as well.

Talk about pleasant projects that the patient will be involved in, together with the family, in the future. Discuss the patient's hobbies and other activities he or she likes.

While the physician cannot predict the future of a patient, you should be aware—and he or she will tell you—that the majority of patients with heart attacks leave the hospital alive, improved, and usually ready soon thereafter to resume their lives.

Heart disease is a serious disease. But there is ample reason for hope, and you should be optimistic. You are very important to the patient while he or she is in the hospital, and your importance will increase when the patient rejoins the family. You have a significant role to play in recovery.

You and your family should attend classes of the local chapter of the American Heart Association to learn the technique of cardiopulmonary resuscitation (CPR). Even if you never have to use this knowledge, it will make you and the patient feel better knowing that you may be able to save the patient's—or someone else's—life if called upon to do so.

How Can I Help a Person Who Appears to Be Having a Heart Attack?

If someone complains of a heart attack or shows symptoms of one—such as severe chest pain, perhaps with pain radiating to arm, jaw, or back, often accompanied by short-windedness, heartbeat disturbance, ashen gray face, and perspiration—prompt action is necessary. Sometimes the victim may be unconscious, in a faint, or the symptoms may be difficult for you to interpret accurately. No matter. If you have any reason at all to think that it may be a heart attack, don't lose time—but don't panic.

Get help as quickly as possible: call an ambulance or the fire department rescue squad. In some places, there is a special telephone number for such emergencies.

When a telephone call is impossible, take the victim as quickly as possible to the nearest hospital emergency room.

While there is little you can do to help the victim directly in such circumstances if you have no special training, you can help by being sure that there are no obstructions in the mouth or at the throat that might inhibit breathing.

If you are skilled in cardiopulmonary resuscitation (CPR) you should use your training.

What Precisely Is Involved in Cardiopulmonary Resuscitation?

It is a relatively simple procedure to learn. It is best learned, as I've indicated, by attending an American Heart Association or other duly organized class, rather than from a book.

CPR is meant to be used under certain circumstances, while waiting for ambulance or rescue squad to appear.

Usually, a victim requiring CPR has had an arrest of heartbeat and breathing. And CPR involves artificial respiration and external cardiac compression to restore both. Quickness, coolness, and determination are essential.

CPR is best managed by two people, one to administer artificial respiration and the other to apply external cardiac compression. If one person must do both jobs, it is difficult but not impossible.

The patient should be stretched out; face up, on a hard surface such as the floor; a bed or couch will not do unless some firm object is placed under the victim's back.

Tilt the chin upward, as shown in Figure 1. Make certain that the mouth and throat contain no obstructions. If any are present, clear them.

Pinch the nostrils shut so no air will escape when you blow into the mouth (see Fig. 2).

Blow into the mouth at a rate of not less than twelve breaths a minute, or once every five seconds (for a child, even more often, once every three seconds). You can determine seconds by counting "one thousand, two thousand, three thousand, four thousand, five thousand"—which makes five seconds.

Each time you blow, the patient's chest will expand moderately. If it fails to do so, there is probably some obstruction, which you should immediately clear from the mouth or throat. After each breath, take your mouth away to permit air to be exhaled.

You should maintain this artificial respiration regularly and rhythmically until the patient is breathing or until help arrives.

Meanwhile, ideally, the other rescuer will be applying cardiac compression. No coordination of your two efforts is required.

For cardiac compression, one palm is placed on the lower end of the patient's breastbone. The other hand is placed on top of and at a right angle to the first.

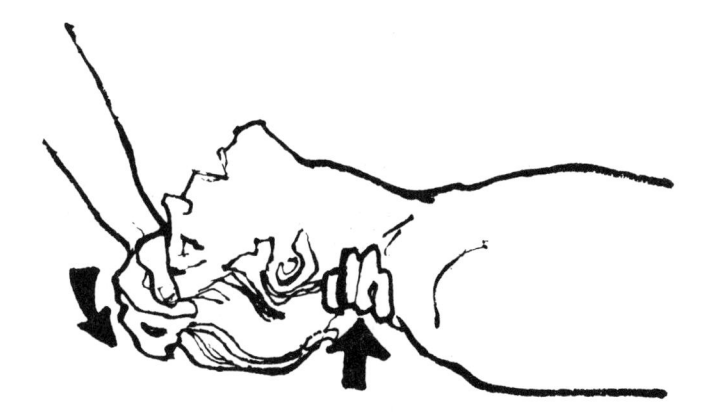

Figure 1. Head-tilt method of opening airway

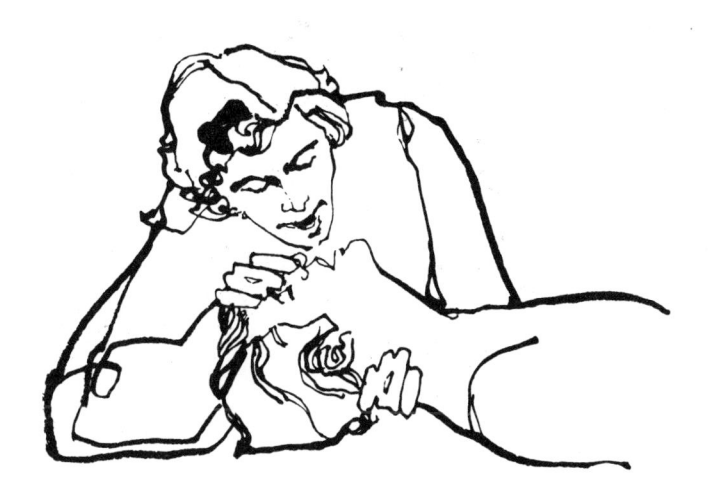

Figure 2. Mouth-to-mouth resuscitation

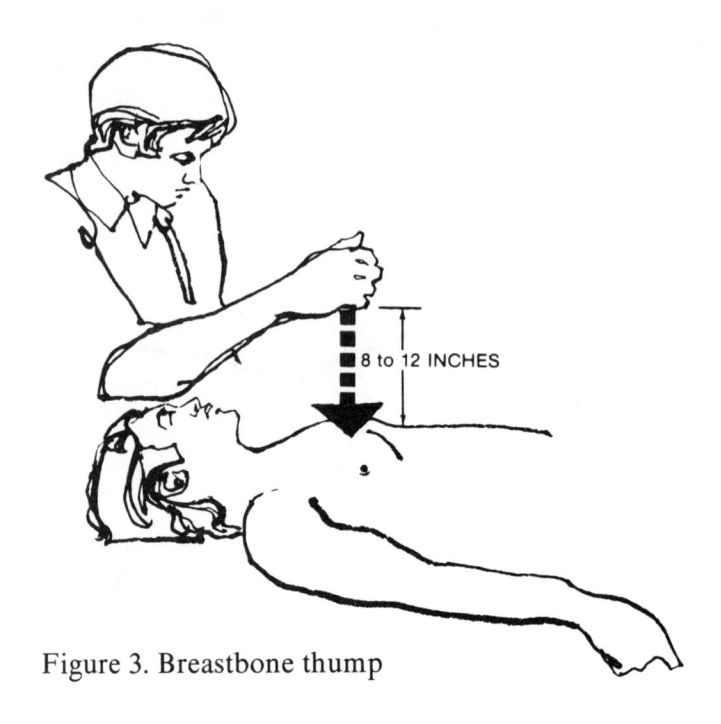

Figure 3. Breastbone thump

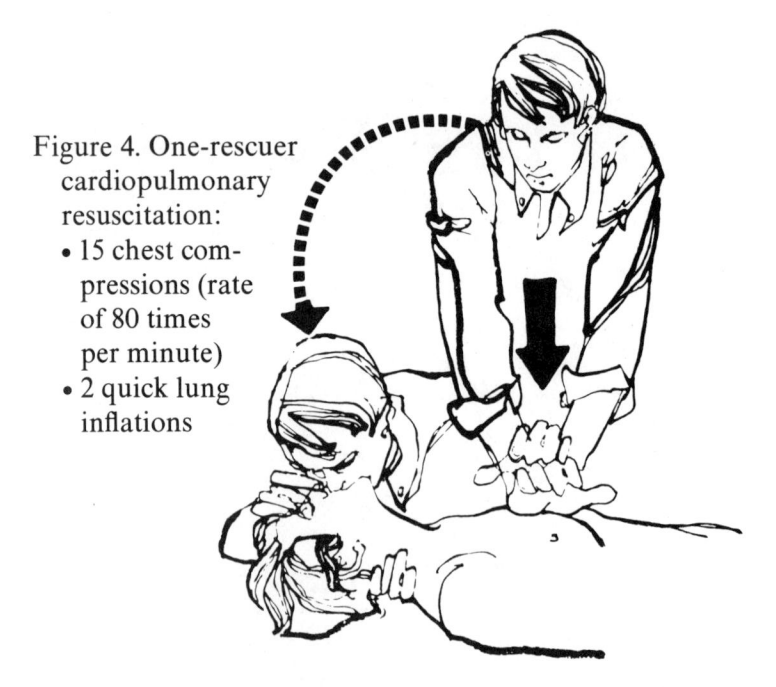

Figure 4. One-rescuer cardiopulmonary resuscitation:
- 15 chest compressions (rate of 80 times per minute)
- 2 quick lung inflations

The rescuer then puts his full weight on his hands, keeping both arms stiff in a steady rhythm of 60 to 70 times a minute. For small children, the rate should be 80 to 100 per minute and only the heel of one hand is used. For infants use only the tips of the index and middle fingers.

The breastbone will move down about two inches or a little less. If you witness a cardiac arrest and if there is no response by the patient within one minute to cardiac compression, try a sharp blow on the breastbone, using your fist and thumping it down from a distance of about eight to twelve inches, as indicated in Figure 3. This may help to restore a normal heart rhythm. In any case, continue cardiac compression until help arrives.

If you yourself have to do both compression and artificial respiration, remember that breathing comes first. Apply artificial respiration first for five breaths, then go to cardiac compression. Establish a pattern of two quick breaths after each fifteen cardiac compressions (see Fig. 4). Never delay compression for longer than five seconds.

If you are alone you should compress the chest at a faster rate, 80 compressions per minute, in order to achieve an actual rate of 60 per minute. The faster rate is necessary to compensate for the lost time the single rescuer needs for the lung inflations.

If I Have a Heart Attack During Work, Am I Entitled to Compensation?

The laws vary from state to state. They also differ for different occupations. Thus, there is no single answer to this question.

Should you have any doubt, check with the local office of the compensation commissioner. Frequently, decisions on the liability of an employer require lengthy court trials, usually between an insurance company and the patient claiming compensation. You may wish to seek the advice of a lawyer or of the local legal aid office.

Most laws provide that any heart attack suffered during, or within a reasonable period after, an unusual physical exertion or mental strain at work will be compensated. It is presumed that in some way these situations precipitated the heart attack. It is not necessarily critical that heart disease did or did not exist prior to the heart attack.

Some employees—for example, members of the armed forces and police and fire departments—usually receive compensation for a heart attack if no hypertension or heart disease was found at the pre-employment medical examination. If you are an employee of private industry, compensation may be more difficult to get.

If you have a heart attack and are unable to work, there are special forms of compensation under Social Security, usually after six months of disability.

What Kind of Physician Should I Choose If I Have Risk Factors for Heart Disease or Already Suffer from Heart Disease?

You should maintain contact with your primary physician—that is, your family physician (general practitioner) or your internist, whether or not you belong to a high-risk group. This physician, of course, should be competent and responsible, keep up with progress in medicine, and know his or her limitations.

If you belong to a high-risk group, a consultation with a cardiologist is advisable. Your primary physician should be made aware of the conclusions of any consultation. The cardiologist is not usually best equipped to be your primary physician. The cardiologist is trained to concentrate upon the cardiovascular system and you may have problems that have nothing to do with your heart. A well-qualified general physician or internist, trained to care for your total well-being, is preferable, provided that he or she works together with your cardiologist as necessary.

Should you have any difficulty finding a primary physician, the local medical society or the medical director of a nearby hospital may be helpful.

If I Have a Heart Attack at an Early Age or If I Have Many Risk Factors, How Can I Prevent Heart Disease in My Children?

As a parent, you should realize, as you seem to, that your children are likely to be prone to the disease, given your heart disease history or propensity. You should discuss this with your physician.

If you do not yet have children, your discussion may help you determine whether to have children or whether adoption may make more sense for you. Your physician may be able to reassure you that the risk for your children is not likely to be great and that it may be compensated for by attention to any risk factors they may have.

If you already have children, you should do everything possible to educate them about risk factors and the need for reducing or eliminating them.

While it is not advisable to test all babies and children routinely for possible high blood fat levels, such tests should be performed if one or both parents belongs to the high-risk group or has had a heart attack at an early age. Should the test show high levels, proper treatment can be initiated by the pediatrician during childhood.

Some physicians believe that a cholesterol test is not always reliable in an infant. It is also possible that a low-cholesterol diet might interfere with early brain development for which cholesterol is necessary.

Therefore, many physicians advise no alterations in diet until a child is at least four years of age, when brain development is completed and tests are more reliable.

Any medication should be kept to a minimum. The reduction of cholesterol and excess fats in a child's diet should come about naturally through the family diet. That is, you will be on a low-cholesterol, moderated fat, and low-sugar diet and, if indicated, the whole family should be on the same diet. Learning about diet in childhood has been shown to have a strong influence on diet in later years. Your children will be grateful to have learned from you that foods can taste good without having to be loaded with cholesterol, excessive amounts of fats, or sugar.

Any further measures to decrease risk factors in a child should be individualized for the child by a pediatrician or a special clinic.

As children grow up, they should be shown, by example, the importance of sticking to a good diet, of leading a physically active life, of not smoking, and of drinking little or no alcohol (particularly if blood triglycerides are elevated). Children can learn, by example in the family, to avoid excess weight and to maintain useful contact with the family physician. In short, they can learn the elements of a healthy life.

If you smoke, you should stop for the sake of your children as well as your own. The best instruction you can give them about smoking is by your own example, coupled with your explanation of the medical reasons why you don't smoke.

Every high school student should have a thorough medical examination at some point before graduation. Be sure that this examination includes measurement of blood pressure and tests to determine the levels of cholesterol, triglycerides, uric acid, and blood sugar. These are simple tests, and the information they provide can do much to help assure a healthy life for your child.

At no time should concern about heart disease become an obsession; that may badly influence the quality of life of parents and children alike.

It is simply a matter of recognizing realities—of reasonable effort to be aware of any risks and to avoid, eliminate, or minimize them.

Is Heart Failure the Same as a Heart Attack?

No, it is not.

While heart failure may occasionally be caused by a heart attack, it may also result from high blood pressure, congenital heart disease, viral infection, changes in heart rhythm, rheumatic fever, physical injury to the heart, or too much alcohol.

In heart failure, the heart does not stop beating. Rather, pumping efficiency is impaired.

One or both ventricles, or pumping chambers, of the heart

may be affected. Should the left ventricle fail, it pumps some blood out into the aorta to be circulated to the body, but some blood remains behind. The left atrium, then, must work harder to move blood into the left ventricle, and pressure within both the atrium and ventricle increases. After a time, the atrium accumulates an excess of blood, and the increased pressure in the atrium is transmitted backward to the pulmonary vein, which transports blood from the lungs to the atrium. Excess blood then accumulates in the lungs. And with the lung congestion, the patient experiences shortness of breath and may wheeze and cough up foamy sputum.

Meanwhile, the left ventricle's inability to pump out adequate blood into the aorta and to the body affects the kidneys, impairing their function. Urine output then drops, and not enough fluid is removed from the blood by the kidneys. The retention of water in the blood increases blood volume and adds to congestion in the lungs.

Should the right ventricle also fail it may stretch, and the right atrium then must work harder to fill the enlarged ventricle. This increases pressure in the atrium and the pressure is transmitted backward through the vein system, which leads to interference with return of used blood from the tissues. Fluid then accumulates in and swells the ankles, the legs, and the abdomen.

Acute failure of either side of the heart, or of course of both sides, requires urgent treatment, which is usually successful.

What Is the Treatment for Heart Failure?

Treatment will include rest, which is important because it helps to reduce the heart's work load. Digitalis may be used to increase pumping efficiency. Restricted salt intake may be prescribed, along with diuretic drugs, to rid the body of excess fluids. Fluid retention usually responds to diuretic and dietary treatment. If the response is not entirely satisfactory, and when excess fluid in the abdominal and chest cavities increases breathing difficulty, the fluid may be removed by needle.

After heart failure has been overcome, measures may be

used to help assure that it does not recur. These will vary with the individual patient and the cause of the heart failure. In some cases, small doses of digitalis will be continued. Other medication may be required—for controlling high blood pressure if that is a problem. In some cases, continued restriction of salt and fluid intake may be advisable.

In heart failure due to a heart attack, careful treatment for several weeks is usually required to give the heart a chance to form a firm scar and for the heart muscle to regain strength and proper function.

10

Frontiers

Coronary heart disease, of course, is no newcomer among diseases. It undoubtedly affected people many millennia ago. Not until 1912, when a Chicago physician, Dr. J. B. Herrick, put all the pieces of evidence together, was the concept of acute coronary thrombosis arrived at in this country. Even then, little was known about the mechanism of the disease beyond the heart attack.

We have come a long way in our understanding in recent years. Almost certainly, further progress can be expected—some of it quite likely within a very few years. In this chapter, I would like to tell you of some of the promising work now going on. Much of it is in relatively early stages—and it is to be expected that some of it will prove invalid or of little or no practical value. I emphasize this because I do not wish to raise false hopes.

On the other hand, I want you to know that intensive research is going on and that some of the efforts are likely to prove rewarding, a few of them perhaps within a few years, so that you or a loved one may be a beneficiary.

Why Is Heart Disease Mortality Declining?

In very recent years, the heart disease mortality rate has declined strikingly. There are still too many deaths—but the numbers were expected to increase, not decrease.

Between 1950 and 1963 coronary mortality increased by 19 percent and peaked in 1963. It started to decline in 1964 and by 1967 was clearly declining for every decade of life. The reduction between 1963 and 1967 was only slight, but that represented a remarkable change from the consistent increase before that. And in recent years, the rate of decline has accelerated.

All told, between 1963 and 1975, the last year for which complete figures are available, these were the declines by age-groups:

>For ages 35 through 44—27.2%
>>ages 45 through 54—27.4%
>>ages 55 through 64—23.5%
>>ages 65 through 74—25.3%
>>ages 75 through 84—12.8%
>>ages 85 and above—19.3%

What was going on?

In January 1964 the surgeon general of the U.S. Public Health Service warned of the health hazards of tobacco consumption, particularly cigarette smoking. A few months later the American Heart Association recommended a change in the general American diet, with the specific goal of reducing heart attacks and strokes by limiting intake of saturated fat and cholesterol.

And between 1963 and 1975, although the overall consumption of some of these products has increased because of the increase in population, there has been an actual decline in per capita consumption of tobacco, animal fats and oils, butter, liquid milk, cream, and eggs, with an associated increase in consumption of vegetable fats and oils. These were the changes:

All tobacco products	22.4% decline
Fluid milk and cream	19.2% decline
Butter	31.9% decline
Eggs	12.0% decline
Animal fats and oils	56.7% decline
Vegetable fats and oils	44.1% increase

The fact that events occur together does not necessarily mean that one may be the cause of the other. But that possibility is not excluded.

If a change in eating and smoking habits—perhaps aided by greater attention to other risk factors such as high blood pressure and what appears to be a marked increase in physical activities—caused or contributed to the encouraging, even remarkable, downward shift in the trend of coronary mortality, further change should accelerate this.

It had been thought, somewhat disconsolately, by some physicians that it was too much to expect any real change in life-style from a population of more than 200 million people.

Yet, obviously, and very hopefully, the American public has demonstrated the ability to change.

Can Artery Disease—Atherosclerosis—Be Reversed?

There is some recent evidence that this *may* be possible.

At the University of Chicago, investigators fed monkeys high-cholesterol diets for eighteen months, then sacrificed some of the animals and on autopsy found extensive coronary artery and other artery disease.

They then divided the remaining monkeys into two groups, one group remaining on the high-cholesterol and high-fat diet, the other placed on a low-cholesterol, low-fat diet. Later, upon sacrifice, the animals on the low-cholesterol, low-fat diet were found to have markedly fewer deposits on their artery linings than did the others, suggesting to the two investigators that "to some degree, even advanced stages of the disease can be reversed if sufficiently low blood cholesterol levels are sustained for a long period of time."

More recently, a study with humans was reported in the February 1977 issue of the *Annals of Internal Medicine* by a team of University of Southern California investigators. In the California study twenty-five patients participated, ranging in age from twenty-two to sixty-five. All had high blood fat levels and many had high blood pressure.

The patients were treated for thirteen months to get the blood fat levels down and, where necessary, to lower elevated blood pressure. A sensitive new radiographic technique was used before and after the study to view the femoral (thigh) arteries and indications in them of atherosclerotic disease.

In nine patients, there were signs of regression of atherosclerotic plaques in the arteries—and in all nine, and only in those nine, there was significant lowering of blood fat levels and elevated pressure. Lack of significant lowering in the other sixteen patients may have resulted from failure of some to comply with treatment or possibly a lack of effectiveness of the particular treatment in their cases.

The California scientists caution that their findings in a small number of patients "should not be interpreted too broadly." Their study does not indicate whether treatment of elevated blood fat levels and hypertension will improve more advanced atherosclerosis. "Nonetheless," they say, "it seems encouraging that *early* human atherosclerosis...can show improvement when patients are treated."

Are the findings, as far as they go, applicable to the coronary arteries, not just the femoral? The investigators believe so, but they note that confirmation will require development of a technique to measure severity of coronary atherosclerosis with the same precision and sensitivity possible in the simple, straight, relatively motionless femoral artery.

Can Elimination of Smoking Lead to Reversal of Atherosclerosis?

In an extension of their work, the same University of Southern California investigating team has reported very early, preliminary evidence of regression of atherosclerotic plaques in the femoral arteries of heart patients who have stopped smoking.

In describing their studies, the scientists emphasize that their findings are very preliminary and incomplete, and that substantial follow-up will be necessary.

Are There Any Important Promising New Insights into Blood Fat Levels?

Yes there are, from recent studies.

Fatty materials like cholesterol don't mix with water, of course. So the blood can't transport them as such. In order to carry the fats, the body hooks them onto proteins that dissolve in the blood serum. Since fats are known as lipids, the fat-protein combinations are called lipoproteins.

As discussed earlier, there is an emerging theory that one type of lipoprotein, called low-density lipoprotein, is the form in which cholesterol is carried to the cells. The evidence is less clear, but it seems that a second type, called high-density lipoprotein, may be what clears and transports cholesterol out of the cells.

Recently, researchers who have been monitoring heart disease for decades in the Framingham Study issued a somewhat startling report. They had found in the latest investigations what was well known, that people with excessive cholesterol in the form of low-density lipoproteins have the greatest risk of heart attack. But they had also found that if the excessive cholesterol was in high-density lipoproteins, the people seemed to be protected against heart attack.

So far the research has been largely limited to people over age fifty. Whether the same distinction holds for younger people remains to be studied.

The immediate implication of the finding is that in older people, at least, excessive amounts of cholesterol in the form of low-density lipoproteins are what need to be treated—but if the cholesterol is high-density lipoprotein, "these people don't need treatment. They're really better off than most people in the U.S." according to the Framingham Study.

It's certain that much new research will be devoted to these findings—and, of course, to the question; If high-density lipoprotein is so good for you, how can you raise your levels of it?

There is only a little documented evidence thus far about how this can be done, but a group of researchers in New Orleans has shown that getting people to run will raise their levels of high-density lipoproteins.

The Framingham Study also indicates that a change of diet can have a similar effect. The diet that brings up the high-density lipoprotein level is one resembling the typical Asian or Mediterranean diet, one that emphasizes vegetables, cereals, fish, little if any meat, and no "junk foods" like hot dogs or potato chips that are packed with saturated fats. The Framingham Study also underscores the importance of diets low in salt and nitrites.

When a Heart Attack Occurs, Can Heart Muscle Damage Be Limited?

Among patients hospitalized with heart attacks, there have been two principal causes of death, when death occurs.

One cause has been abnormal heart rhythm, and deaths from this have been greatly reduced in recent years through use of modern monitoring techniques in the coronary care unit and the use of anti-arrhythmic drugs and other measures.

The second cause has been and remains pump failure. Some heart attack victims who survive the initial damage in the first minutes after an attack die a few days later because of pump failure resulting from destruction of a large amount of heart muscle—and mortality due to pump failure has shown little change in recent years.

Such pump failure, some investigators believe, occurs when initial damage to the heart continues to spread for hours or even days after the attack until it becomes so extensive that the heart is no longer able to function. Studies are now under way to find methods of keeping the damage from spreading.

The work is in early stages and no firm conclusions can be drawn yet; it may be several years before any can be. But it is clearly work of potentially great importance.

In one study, for example, investigators of Peter Bent Brigham Hospital and Harvard Medical School in Boston, Massachusetts, have worked with a drug, hyaluronidase. The drug was chosen because it improves the spread of other substances throughout the body and is sometimes used to increase the spread of injected drugs. Theoretically, it might improve the spread of oxygen and nutrients to the sections of heart muscle that are endangered by the heart attack and thus possibly keep them alive. And recent animal experiments have suggested that hyaluronidase can limit the spread of damage to the heart muscle.

In the Boston study the research team compared the electrocardiograms of forty-six heart attack victims who had been treated with hyaluronidase by injection with the ECGs of forty-five patients who received conventional treatment for their heart attacks.

The drug, which was administered within eight hours after the heart attack, did not "cure" the initial damage of the heart attack, but the electrocardiographic evidence indicates that the amount of damage in the treated patients was less extensive than in those not receiving the drug.

The report of the study emphasizes that the number of heart attack patients involved is not large enough to determine whether damage limitation following a heart attack will increase the chances of survival or of faster recovery. A new federally financed, large-scale study of such treatment is planned to assess the effects on mortality of heart patients.

Are We Ever Likely to Have a Practical Artificial Heart?

Many serious investigators in Houston and Boston believe so and are working to develop one. The problems in doing so are extremely difficult but not necessarily insurmountable.

An artificial heart would be a mechanical device, a pump, to maintain circulation. That this is not impossible has been demonstrated, of course, by the success of the heart-lung machine.

Several prototype artificial heart models have been developed. One, for example, is made up of two air-driven pumps made of plastic, with flexible rubber bladders. The device, with its pumps that would replace the ventricles or pumping chambers of the natural heart, might be attached to remnants of the upper chambers of the heart. Pumping would be achieved by introduction of air to collapse the bladders and force blood out, with the beat of the device triggered by pacemaking cells in the remnant of the upper right atrium of the natural heart. Impulses from the pacemaking cells would be amplified electronically.

Another prototype, working on a similar principle, has two silicone collapsible ventricles inside a rigid plastic housing and also uses an electronic device to control beating.

Such models, and others—which have been used experimentally in animals—get their power from consoles outside the body. And one need that must be met is for an implantable power source. For this, various possibilities have been under study, including devices that could convert body heat to electricity and others that could convert body motion into electricity. A nuclear-powered battery is a possibility.

But still other problems remain. When blood is in long contact with any surface other than the lining of blood vessels and the natural heart, it undergoes gradual destruction of important elements. A suitable material to line the artificial heart must be found—no easy matter since it must be accepted and not rejected by the body, must not cause allergic or toxic reactions, and must be strong enough to withstand stress for many years.

Difficult as these problems are, many researchers believe they can be solved, possibly within the next decade.

When If Ever Will Heart Transplants Become Practical?

No one can say. Progress has been made—and hard-won. Much yet remains to be made, even disregarding the problem of donation.

In the first ten years, since the first heart transplant was done in 1967, there have been, throughout the world, 333 heart transplants on 325 patients. As this is written, 69 persons still survive, the longest survivor being a Frenchman who received his new heart in Marseilles, France, on November 26, 1968.

Initially there was great enthusiasm for the procedure; later optimism slackened. By 1974, for example, only 27 heart transplants were performed, 15 of them by a team at Stanford University School of Medicine. After eight years, the Stanford team could report their experience with 90 transplants, with 32 still alive and the longest survivor having lived 5⅔ years.

Survival rates for the entire series of patients were 47 percent after one year and 37 percent after three years. For those 53 patients surviving the critical first three postoperative months, these figures rose to 76 percent and 59 percent respectively.

In the report, which was presented at the 48th Annual Scientific Sessions of the American Heart Association, the Stanford team compared patients receiving heart transplants with those dying before donors became available, demonstrating a much improved survival rate for those getting new hearts. The average time period between selection as a candidate for transplantation and the operation was thirty-five days as compared to a forty-seven-day interval between selection and death when a donor was not available. These very similar time periods make it unlikely that only sicker patients died before surgery, the report added: "Thus, we feel certain that transplantation increases the length of survival in our carefully selected group of patients."

The criteria for patient selection are rigorous. To be selected, a patient's disease must be so severe that he or she is limited to a bed-to-chair existence, and no further medical or surgical treatment is possible. Many patients selected, usually under fifty years of age, have required frequent rehospitalization before, and all have had a clinically estimated life span of less than six months without heart transplantation.

According to the Stanford report, heart transplantation "clearly improves the quality of life in surviving patients." Of the fifty-three once-bedridden or otherwise-severely-limited patients, forty-eight (91 percent) could return to "normal activity status"—meaning no symptoms even with vigorous activity. Forty of the forty-eight returned to their previous occupation or activities; eight retired voluntarily.

Survivors of the operation required an average of seventy-two days of hospitalization—and in-patient costs for the operation and early postoperative care have averaged $36,130 per patient.

From the beginning of transplant operations, a major

problem has been rejection—the body's blind effort to throw off the new heart, vital as it is, because it is foreign. Better methods of matching donor heart to patient and refinement of methods of combating rejection have helped. But rejection is still a recurrent problem, though not a major cause of death in long-term survivors. (New techniques of early recognition and treatment of rejection also help improve outlook.)

Susceptibility to infection, however, has remained, thus far, an inevitable side effect of the treatments used to suppress the body's immune system, which causes rejection but also fights off infection. Infections have become the major cause of death in long-term survivors.

Will further progress be made? Undoubtedly.

How long before heart transplantation can become practical on a large scale—considering problems of obtaining adequate numbers of donor hearts to assure the best possible matching with potential recipients, problems of rejection and infection, and problems of cost? At this time we do not know.

11

A Parting Word

As you have read the questions and answers I have taken up, perhaps some answers have left you pessimistic and others have left you confused. But there is no real cause for either pessimism or confusion.

Yes, there do remain some aspects of atherosclerosis, coronary heart disease, and heart attacks that need more light thrown upon them. And there are controversies among experts in some areas.

Yet the fact is that while the disease is common and dangerous the mortality from it has been decreasing. Keep in mind that of the many patients with coronary heart disease now more remain alive than die from it. And keep in mind, too, that the quality of life for most patients who are surviving has been greatly—remarkably—improved.

As far as treatment goes, it is not static, unmoving, in a rut. It is dynamic, constantly changing and advancing, due to intensive research all over the world.

One of these days the very core of the mechanism of atherosclerotic heart disease may be uncovered and then there may be opportunity to attack it right there, to interrupt the mechanism, and stop the process cold. The disease might then be done away with, completely eliminated.

Meanwhile, much can be done with the tools available today. It is good that there are controversies among experts in some areas. That helps to spur research. It is good that new methods and medications are being introduced almost continuously. And it is good that the experienced, alert physician is neither the first to embrace a new, unproven treatment nor the last to discard an older measure which has proved to be less effective or not effective at all and has become obsolete.

As much as possible, you need to acquire—and will be greatly helped by—a deepening basic understanding of coronary heart disease. And I hope that this book will be helpful in that, particularly with rereading and when used as a reference for any new problem that may arise or perhaps for some new doubt that troubles you.

You need too, very much, a physician you can trust. If you follow his or her advice with greater understanding, occasionally consulting with a cardiologist when and if this is warranted, you may have a good chance to escape heart disease if thus far it has been only a threat. And even if afflicted, you may have a very good chance to survive for a long time—to enjoy life and remain a valuable and valued member of society.

Glossary

ADRENALINE: A secretion of the adrenal glands that lie above the kidneys. It constricts small blood vessels and increases heart rate and blood pressure. Also called epinephrine.

ANGINA PECTORIS: Chest pain or pressure caused by inadequate blood supply to the heart muscle, commonly resulting from narrowing of the coronary arteries that feed the heart muscle. The pain is paroxysmal, usually comes on with effort or excitement, may spread from the chest to jaw, shoulder, and down the left arm, or, rarely, from chest to abdomen and back of chest.

ANGIOCARDIOGRAPHY: An X-ray study of the blood vessels following the injection of an opaque fluid, or dye, into the bloodstream.

ANOXIA: Lack of oxygen, most often the result of complete cutoff of blood supply to a part of the body, such as an area of heart muscle.

ANTICOAGULANT: An agent that slows blood coagulation or clotting.

ANTIHYPERTENSIVE AGENT: A drug that lowers blood pressure.

ANXIETY: An apprehensive feeling, the source of which may not be recognizable.

AORTA: The main trunk artery of the body. It starts at the base of the heart where it receives blood from the heart's left ventricle. Much like the handle of a cane, the aorta arches up over the heart, then extends down through the chest and abdomen in front of the spine. Many arteries branch off at various points from the aorta to carry blood to various body areas, including the heart muscle.

ARRHYTHMIA: An abnormal heartbeat.

ARTERIOSCLEROSIS: Hardening of the arteries. A term that covers various conditions that cause artery walls to thicken, harden, and lose their elasticity. *See* ATHEROSCLEROSIS.

ARTERY: A blood vessel that carries oxygen-rich blood away from the heart to some area of the body.

ATHEROMA: A deposit of fat and other substances in the inner lining of an artery.

ATHEROSCLEROSIS: A kind of arteriosclerosis in which deposits of fatty materials (atheromata, plural of atheroma) are laid down in the inner layer of an artery wall, making the wall thick and irregular and projecting so that the internal diameter of the artery is decreased.

ATRIUM (plural: ATRIA): An upper chamber of the heart. The right atrium receives blood returning from the body; the left atrium receives fresh, richly oxygenated blood from the lungs.

AURICLE: Another name for ATRIUM.

AUSCULTATION: Listening, usually with a stethoscope, to sounds within the body.

AUTONOMIC NERVOUS SYSTEM: The system—sometimes also called the involuntary or vegetative nervous system—that controls the workings of such organs and tissues as the heart, glands, and smooth muscles.

BACTERIAL ENDOCARDITIS: A bacteria-caused inflammation of the heart's inner lining or the lining of the heart

GLOSSARY

valves. Most often, it results from infection elsewhere in the body, from an operation, or from injury.

BLOOD LIPIDS: Fat or fatlike substances in the blood, including triglycerides and cholesterol.

BLOOD PLATELETS: Round or oval disks in the blood that play an important role in blood coagulation or clotting. When a small blood vessel is injured, platelets adhere to each other and to the edges of the injury, forming a plug or clot that covers the area and stops loss of blood.

BLOOD PRESSURE: The pressure of blood in the arteries. The greater pressure, which comes when the heart contracts (systole) is called systolic pressure; the pressure between beats, when the heart is relaxed (diastole), is called diastolic.

BRADYCARDIA: An abnormally slow heartbeat rate—below 60 beats per minute in an adult or below 70 in a child.

BRADY-TACHYCARDIA: A heart rhythm disorder in which the heart beats too slowly at times, too rapidly at other times.

BYPASS SURGERY: An operation in which a partially or completely blocked portion of an artery is bypassed, or detoured around, through use of a section of vein or another artery from the patient, so that an adequate blood supply may reach areas previously deprived of it.

CARDIAC: Relating to the heart. The plural is sometimes used to refer to people who have heart disease.

CARDIAC OUTPUT: The amount of blood pumped by the heart in one minute.

CARDIOVASCULAR: Relating to the heart and blood vessels.

CARDITIS: Inflammation of the heart.

CATHETER: A thin tube of plastic or other material that can be inserted into a vein or artery or other orifice of the body.

CATHETERIZATION, CARDIAC: The use of a catheter to

examine the heart. The catheter is usually introduced into a vein or artery in the arm and moved into the heart where it may be used to take pressure readings or blood samples for study.

CIRCULATORY: Relating to the heart, blood vessels, and circulation of blood.

CLAUDICATION: Leg pain and limping or lameness resulting from inadequate circulation in leg blood vessels because of atherosclerosis.

COAGULATION: The conversion of a liquid to a thick or solid material; formation of a blood clot.

COARCTATION OF THE AORTA: A constriction or narrowing of the aorta, the trunk artery of the body.

COLLATERAL CIRCULATION: The circulation of blood through nearby small accessory blood vessels when a main vessel or branch becomes blocked.

CONGESTIVE HEART FAILURE: A condition in which congestion, or fluid accumulation, occurs in various parts of the body, such as lungs, legs, abdomen, when the heart cannot pump out effectively all the blood that returns to it.

CORONARY ARTERIES: The two arteries that come off the aorta, or main trunk-line artery, and arch down over the heart to carry blood to the heart muscle.

CORONARY ATHEROSCLEROSIS: A thickening with deposits on the walls of the coronary arteries so that the channel through which blood flows is narrowed, reducing the flow. Also called coronary artery disease and coronary heart disease.

CORONARY OCCLUSION: Obstruction of a coronary artery or branch, impeding blood flow to part of the heart muscle. Sometimes called coronary thrombosis. Also called heart attack.

CORONARY THROMBOSIS: Formation of a clot that blocks a coronary artery or branch.

DEFIBRILLATOR: Any measure, such as a device that pro-

GLOSSARY

duces an electric shock, to stop fibrillation or useless, uncoordinated heart muscle contraction and restore normal heartbeat.

DIASTOLE: The period when the heart relaxes between beats.

DIASTOLIC BLOOD PRESSURE: The pressure measurement in between beats of the heart. Recorded as the lower figure in a blood pressure reading such as the 80 in 120/80.

DIGITALIS: A drug derived from the leaves of the foxglove and capable of strengthening heart contractions and slowing the contraction rate, improving heart efficiency.

DILATION: Enlargement of the heart or blood vessels.

DIURESIS: Increased excretion of urine.

DIURETIC: A drug that promotes increased urine excretion.

DYSPNEA: Difficult or labored breathing.

ECHOCARDIOGRAPHY: The sending of ultrasonic waves through the heart and the recording of the reflection of the waves to permit diagnosis of various heart abnormalities.

ELECTROCARDIOGRAM: A record, also called ECG and EKG, of electric currents produced by the heart, useful in diagnosis of various heart abnormalities.

ELECTROCARDIOGRAM, HOLTER: A continuous electrocardiogram recorded on a portable instrument while the patient moves around during daily activities.

ELECTROCARDIOGRAPH: An instrument for recording the heart's electric current.

EMBOLISM: The obstruction of a blood vessel by a clot or other material carried to the site in the bloodstream from elsewhere.

EMBOLUS: A clot or other material such as fat or air carried in the blood to a small vessel where it becomes lodged and impedes blood flow.

ENDOCARDITIS: Inflammation of the heart's inner lining, or

endocardium, usually resulting from rheumatic fever or infection.

ENZYME: One of a group of complex chemicals, of which the body has many, that speed up biochemical processes.

EPINEPHRINE: A secretion of the adrenal glands that lie above the kidneys, which constricts small blood vessels, and increases the pulse rate and blood pressure. Also called adrenaline.

ERYTHROCYTE: A red blood cell. It contains hemoglobin, a pigment that gives it its color and also transports oxygen and carbon dioxide.

ESSENTIAL HYPERTENSION: High blood pressure for which there is no known organic cause.

ETIOLOGY: The science dealing with the causes of disease.

EXTRACORPOREAL CIRCULATION: Circulation of the blood outside the body, as by a heart-lung machine during heart surgery.

EXTRASYSTOLE: A premature heart contraction that interrupts normal heart rhythm.

EYEGROUND: The inside of the back portion of the eye, which can be seen through the pupil with an instrument, the ophthalmoscope. Its examination is helpful in assessing changes in blood vessels. Also called the fundus.

FIBRILLATION: Contractions of the heart that are uncoordinated and amount virtually to mere useless twitchings.

FIBRIN: A material that forms part of a blood clot.

FLUOROSCOPE: An instrument that directs X rays through the body onto a fluorescent screen where shadows of internal organs can be seen.

FUNDUS: *See* EYEGROUND.

GOUT: A disorder of body metabolism or handling of substances called purines that are found in certain high-protein foods. It leads to the appearance of excessive quantities of uric

GLOSSARY

acid in the blood, which may be deposited in the joints and other tissues, causing swelling, inflammation, and extreme pain in a joint.

HEART BLOCK: Interference with the conduction of electrical impulses of the heart so that the atria and ventricles contract independently instead of in coordinated fashion, thus interfering with the rate or regularity of the heartbeat.

HEART-LUNG MACHINE: A machine that both pumps and adds oxygen to the blood so that blood can be diverted from the heart during surgery.

HEART SHOCK: A condition in which, due to weakness of the heart muscle, blood pressure falls low, urinary output drops, the skin becomes clammy, and the patient becomes confused. Heart shock may be a complication of a heart attack.

HEMOGLOBIN: The oxygen-carrying pigment of the red blood cell.

HEMORRHAGE: Loss of blood from a blood vessel. In an external hemorrhage, blood escapes from the body; in an internal hemorrhage, the blood moves into tissues surrounding the ruptured vessel.

HEPARIN: An anticoagulant drug that helps to keep blood from clotting.

HIGH-RISK GROUP: People who are particularly prone to heart disease because of the presence of risk factors such as high blood pressure, elevated cholesterol, elevated uric acid, obesity, smoking, family history of heart disease at an early age, diabetes, and type-A personality.

HORMONAL SHIELD: The protection apparently provided by the female sex hormone, estrogen, during the child-bearing years against the development of atherosclerosis.

HYPERCHOLESTEROLEMIA, or HYPERCHOLESTEREMIA: An excess of cholesterol in the blood.

HYPERLIPEMIA: An excess of fats, or lipids, in the blood.

HYPERTENSION: Also called high blood pressure.

HYPERTHYROIDISM: Exessive activity of the thyroid gland, which may speed the heart rate and many body processes.

HYPERTROPHY: Enlargement of the heart or another organ or tissue.

HYPOTENSION: Also called low blood pressure.

HYPOTHYROIDISM: Underactivity of the thyroid gland, which may slow the heart rate and many body processes.

HYPOXIA: A less than normal amount of oxygen in body organs and tissues.

IATROGENIC HEART DISEASE: Iatrogenic literally means "produced by the doctor." A patient's belief that he or she has heart disease based on inference from a physician's discussion or actions.

INDERAL: *See* PROPRANOLOL.

INFARCT: An area of tissue damaged or dead as a result of insufficient blood supply. As used in the phrase "myocardial infarct" it refers to a heart muscle area damaged or dead because of insufficient blood flow through a coronary artery that normally supplies the area.

INSUFFICIENCY: Incompetency. In the term "myocardial insufficiency" it means inability of the heart to pump normally.

INTIMA: The innermost layer of a blood vessel.

ISCHEMIA: A localized, usually temporary shortage of blood in some area of the body that may be caused by a constriction or obstruction in a blood vessel supplying that area.

ISCHEMIC PERICARDITIS: A localized inflammation of the sac surrounding the heart, in the area above a part of the heart muscle that has died due to blocking of a coronary artery or one of its branches.

ISOENZYME: One of several forms in which an enzyme may exist in various body tissues.

GLOSSARY

ISOMETRIC EXERCISE: Exercise in which tension of a muscle increases with little or no shortening of the muscle, as in pitting one muscle against another or a muscle against an immovable object such as a wall; also in pushups, weight lifting, pulling or pressing springs.

ISOTONIC EXERCISE: Exercise in which a muscle or group of muscles moves as well as contracts, as in walking, jogging, running, swimming, etc.

LDH: Abbreviation for lactic dehydrogenase, an enzyme released in large amounts by a damaged heart.

LINOLEIC ACID: A component of many unsaturated fats, occurring in oils from many plants.

LIPID: Fat.

LIPOPROTEIN: A complex of fat and protein molecules.

LUMEN: The space, passageway, or channel within a blood vessel or tubular organ.

METABOLISM: All the chemical changes that take place within the body.

MONOUNSATURATED FAT: A fat such as olive oil which is so chemically constituted that it can absorb additional hydrogen, but not as much as a polyunsaturated fat. Such fats in the diet have little effect on blood cholesterol levels.

MYOCARDIAL INFARCTION: Damage or death of an area of the heart muscle (the myocardium) caused by reduced blood supply to the area.

MYOCARDIAL INSUFFICIENCY: Inability of the heart muscle to maintain normal circulation.

MYOCARDITIS: Inflammation of the heart muscle.

MYOCARDIUM: The muscular wall of the heart.

NECROSIS: Death of areas of tissue or bone as the result of disease or injury.

NEUROGENIC: Originating in the nervous system.

NITROGLYCERIN: A drug that relaxes the muscles in blood vessels, dilating or expanding the vessels. Often used to relieve or help prevent attacks of angina pectoris.

NORMOTENSIVE: Characterized by normal blood pressure.

NUCLEAR SCANNING: A diagnostic technique in which radioactive material is injected into the bloodstream and is absorbed by the heart muscle. Because absorption of healthy muscle differs from that of diseased muscle, the size of a diseased muscle area can be determined.

OCCLUSION: The act of closure or state of being closed. In coronary occlusion, a coronary vessel becomes occluded because of obstruction by a clot or as the result of spasm.

OPEN-HEART SURGERY: Surgery performed on the opened heart while blood is diverted through a heart-lung machine.

PACEMAKER: (1) A small mass of special cells in the right upper chamber of the heart which produce the electrical impulses that initiate heart contraction; also called sino-atrial node or S-A node. (2) An electric device that can substitute for the natural pacemaker and control beating of the heart by a series of rhythmic electrical discharges.

PALPITATION: A fluttering of the heart or abnormal rhythm or rate of the heart sensed by an individual.

PARASYMPATHETIC NERVOUS SYSTEM: A part of the autonomic, or involuntary, nervous system. The parasympathetic nerves carry impulses that contract the pupils of the eyes, slow the heart rate, and produce other involuntary reactions.

PAROXYSMAL TACHYCARDIA: An episode of rapid heartbeats that begins and ends suddenly.

PATHOGENESIS: The events leading to development of disease.

PATHOLOGY: The study of the nature of disease and changes in structure and function that disease produces.

Glossary

PERCUSSION: Tapping of the body with the fingers as an aid in diagnosis.

PERICARDIUM: The thin sac that envelops the heart.

PHARMACOLOGY: The science dealing with all aspects of drugs.

PHLEBITIS: Inflammation of a vein, often in the leg.

PLAQUE: A patch; a deposit of predominantly fatty material in the lining of blood vessels occurring in atherosclerosis.

PLASMA: The liquid, cell-free portion of uncoagulated blood. It differs from serum, which is the fluid part of blood obtained after coagulation.

POLYUNSATURATED FAT: A fat so made up chemically that it can absorb additional hydrogen. Such a fat is usually a liquid oil of vegetable origin, such as corn or safflower oil. A diet high in polyunsaturated fat tends to lower blood cholesterol levels.

POST-MYOCARDIAL INFARCTION SYNDROME: Pain on breathing often associated with fever, which may occur in some patients two to six weeks after a heart attack. Harmless but distressing, it is due to inflammation of the sac around the heart (the pericardium) or inflammation of the lungs or sac around the lungs, is self-limited, responds well to cortisone, and may recur. Also called Dressler's syndrome after Dr. William Dressler who first described it.

PRINZMETAL ANGINA: Characterized by chest pain at rest and during sleep and by electrocardiographic changes opposite to those seen in the usual type of angina. Also called angina variant.

PROCAINAMIDE: A drug used to restore regular heart rhythm or to prevent irregular heart rhythm.

PROPHYLAXIS: Preventive treatment.

PROPRANOLOL (*Inderal*): A drug used to treat certain abnormal heart rhythms or to decrease angina or blood pressure.

PSYCHOSOMATIC: Having to do with the influence of mind and emotions upon the functions of the body, especially in terms of disease.

PULMONARY ARTERY: The large artery that transports used, unoxygenated blood from the heart to the lungs; it is the only artery that carries unoxygenated blood.

PULMONARY EMBOLISM: Obstruction of the pulmonary artery or one of its branches caused by a clot that usually has traveled up from a leg vein or less commonly from a vein elsewhere in the body.

PULMONARY VEINS: Four veins, two from each lung, that transport oxygenated blood from the lungs to the heart.

PULSE: The expansion and contraction of an artery, which may be felt with the fingers at the wrist or elsewhere. The artery contractions correspond to contractions of the heart and so are indications of heart action.

RENAL: Relating to the kidney.

RHEUMATIC HEART DISEASE: Damage to the heart, particularly the heart valves, by one or more attacks of rheumatic fever, a disease most frequent in childhood, sometimes occurring a few weeks after streptococcal infection and marked by one or more such symptoms as fever, sore and swollen joints, skin rash, or involuntary muscle twitching (chorea, or Saint Vitus's dance).

RISK FACTORS: Factors that predispose to coronary heart disease, including family history of heart attacks at an early age, obesity, high blood pressure, smoking, type-A personality, high cholesterol and uric acid levels.

SATURATED FAT: A fat so constituted chemically that it cannot take on any more hydrogen; usually a solid fat of animal origin, such as in milk, butter, meat. A diet high in saturated fat tends to increase blood levels of cholesterol.

SCLEROSIS: Hardening.

Glossary

SERUM: The fluid portion of blood remaining after cellular elements have been removed by coagulation; different from plasma, which is the cell-free portion of uncoagulated blood.

SIGN: Any objective evidence of a disease. *See also* SYMPTOM.

SINUS NODE: A small mass of specialized cells in the upper right heart chamber which initiate the electrical impulses that produce contractions of the heart. Also called pacemaker, sino-atrial node, and S-A node.

SKIPPED BEAT: A sensation in which the pause following a premature heartbeat is experienced.

SODIUM: A mineral common in plant and animal tissue. Table salt—sodium chloride—is nearly half sodium. In some heart conditions, the body may retain excessive sodium and water, and sodium intake may be limited and/or a diuretic drug used to increase fluid elimination.

SPHYGMOMANOMETER: An instrument for measuring blood pressure.

STETHOSCOPE: An instrument for listening to sounds within the body.

STRESS TEST: The taking of electrocardiograms when exercise is carried out, the exercise involving climbing a set of stairs, walking a treadmill, or riding a stationary bicycle. Electrocardiograms taken this way may show heart disease when electrocardiograms taken at rest fail to reveal it.

STROKE: Also called cerebrovascular accident, or CVA; involving damage or death to an area of the brain caused by reduced blood supply to that area, which may result from blocking of a vessel by a clot formed locally (cerebral thrombosis) or traveling there from elsewhere in the blood vessel system (cerebral embolism), or by rupture of a blood vessel (cerebral hemorrhage).

SYMPATHETIC NERVOUS SYSTEM: One of two parts (the

other being the parasympathetic nervous system) of the autonomic, or involuntary, nervous system that regulates such tissues and organs as glands, heart, and smooth muscles not under voluntary control.

SYMPTOM: Any subjective evidence of a patient's condition. *See also* SIGN.

SYNCOPE: A faint.

SYNDROME: A set of several symptoms that occur together and are given a collective name.

SYSTOLE: The period of contraction or beating of the heart.

TACHYCARDIA: Abnormally fast heartbeat, usually anything over 100 beats a minute.

TACHYCARDIA, ECTOPIC: Abnormally fast heartbeat originating outside the normal point of origin, the sinus node.

THROMBOPHLEBITIS: Inflammation and clotting in a vein.

THROMBOSIS: Formation or presence of a blood clot (thrombus) inside a blood vessel or the heart.

THROMBUS: A blood clot that forms inside a blood vessel or the heart.

TOXIC: Relating to poison.

TRIGLYCERIDE: A fat in which glycerol is combined with three fatty acids (stearic, oleic, palmitic). Most animal fats are triglycerides, and triglyceride is the usual storage form of fat in the human body.

TYPE-A PERSONALITY: A competitive, aggressive person who creates many deadlines, is impatient in carrying out work, tries to achieve too much, becomes hostile, and seems to be prone to heart disease.

UREMIA: An excess in the blood of waste materials normally excreted by the kidneys in the urine.

VASOCONSTRICTOR: A chemical substance, such as adren-

Glossary

aline, that stimulates the muscles of blood vessels to contract, thus narrowing the passage.

VASODILATOR: An agent, such as nitroglycerin, nitrite, or other chemical compound, that causes relaxation of the muscles of blood vessels.

VEIN: A blood vessel that carries blood from some part of the body back to the heart.

VENA CAVA: The superior vena cava is a large vein carrying blood from the upper body (head, neck, chest) to the heart; the inferior vena cava is a large vein carrying blood from the lower body to the heart.

VENOUS BLOOD: Unoxygenated "used" blood carried by the veins from all parts of the body back to the heart.

VENTRICLE: One of the two lower chambers of the heart. The left ventricle pumps fresh, oxygenated blood through arteries to the body; the right ventricle pumps unoxygenated "used" blood through the pulmonary artery to the lungs for oxygenation.

APPENDIX A

Desirable Weights for Men and Women

Height (in shoes) Feet	Inches	Small frame	Medium frame	Large frame
\multicolumn{5}{c}{MEN}
5	2	116–125	124–133	131–142
5	3	119–128	127–136	133–144
5	4	122–132	130–140	137–149
5	5	126–136	134–144	141–153
5	6	129–139	137–147	145–157
5	7	133–143	141–151	149–162
5	8	136–147	145–160	153–166
5	9	140–151	149–160	157–170
5	10	144–155	153–164	161–175
5	11	148–164	157–168	165–180
6	0	152–164	161–173	169–185
6	1	157–169	166–178	174–190
6	2	163–175	171–184	179–196
6	3	168–180	176–189	184–202
\multicolumn{5}{c}{WOMEN}
4	11	104–111	110–118	117–127
5	0	105–113	112–120	119–129
5	1	107–115	114–122	121–131
5	2	110–118	117–125	124–135
5	3	113–121	120–128	127–138
5	4	116–125	124–132	131–142
5	5	119–128	127–135	133–145
5	6	123–132	130–140	138–150
5	7	126–136	134–144	142–154
5	8	129–139	137–147	145–158
5	9	133–143	141–151	149–162
5	10	136–147	145–155	152–166
5	11	139–150	148–158	155–169

APPENDIX B

Table of Spending Calories

Activity	Calories per hour
REST AND LIGHT ACTIVITY	
Lying down or sleeping	80
Sitting	100
Driving a car	120
Standing	140
Domestic work	180
MODERATE ACTIVITY	
Bicycling (5½ mph)	210
Walking (2½ mph)	210
Gardening	220
Canoeing (2½ mph)	230
Golf	250
Lawn mowing (power mower)	250
Bowling	270
Lawn mowing (hand mower)	270
Fencing	300
Rowboating (2½ mph)	300
Swimming (¼ mph)	300
Walking (3¾ mph)	300
Badminton	350
Horseback riding (trotting)	350
Square dancing	350
Volleyball	350
Roller skating	350
VIGOROUS ACTIVITY	
Table tennis	360
Ditch digging	400
Ice skating (10 mph)	400
Wood chopping or sawing	400
Tennis	420
Water skiing	480
Hill climbing (100 ft. per hour)	490
Skiing (10 mph)	600
Squash and handball	600
Bicycling (13 mph)	660
Scull rowing (race)	840
Running (10 mph)	900

NOTE: The caloric expenditures shown in the above table are for an individual weighing 150 pounds. The heavier the person, the more calories expended in each activity.

APPENDIX C

Cholesterol Content of Common Foods

The tabulation below shows the cholesterol content in milligrams of 100-gram (3½-ounce) portions of common foods:

Beef, raw	70	Ice cream	45
Brains, raw	2,000-plus	Kidney, raw	375
Butter	250	Lamb, raw	70
Caviar or fish roe	300-plus	Lard and animal fat	95
Cheddar cheese	100	Liver, raw	300
Creamed cottage cheese	15	Lobster meat	200
Cream cheese	120	Margarine, vegetable fat	0
Cheese spread	65	Margarine, ⅔ animal fat	65
Chicken, raw	60	Milk, whole	11
Crab	125	Milk, skim	3
Egg whole	550	Mutton	65
Egg white	0	Oysters	200-plus
Egg yolk, fresh	1,500	Pork	70
Egg yolk, frozen	1,280	Shrimp	125
Egg yolk, dried	2,950	Sweetbreads	250
Fish fillet	70	Veal	90
Heart, raw	150		

APPENDIX D

Caloric Content of Foods and Beverages

Foods	Amount	Calories
SOUP		
Bouillon or consommé	1 cup	30
Cream soups	1 cup	150
Split pea	1 cup	200
Vegetable-beef or chicken	1 cup	70
Tomato	1 cup	90
Chicken noodle	1 cup	65
Clam chowder	1 cup	85
MEAT AND FISH		
Beefsteak	3 ounces	300
Roast beef	3 ounces	300
Ground beef	3 ounces	245
Roast leg of lamb	3 ounces	250
Rib lamb chop	1 medium	130
Loin pork chop	1 medium	235
Ham, smoked or boiled	2 slices	240
Bacon	2 strips	100
Frankfurter	5½ × ¾ inches	125
Tongue or kidney	average portion	150
Chicken	6 ounces	190
Turkey	3½ ounces	200
Salami	2 ounces	260
Bologna	4 ounces	260
Veal cutlet (unbreaded)	3 ounces	185
Hamburger patty	3 ounces	245

Foods	Amount	Calories
Beef liver, fried	2 ounces	130
Bluefish, baked	3 ounces	135
Fish sticks, breaded (with fat for frying)	4 ounces	200
Tuna fish, canned, drained	⅖ cup	170
Salmon, drained	⅔ cup	140
Sardines, drained	4 ounces	260
Shrimp, canned	4 to 6	65
Trout	average portion	250
Fish (cod, haddock, mackerel, halibut, white, broiled or baked)	average portion	190
Whole lobster	1 pound	145
VEGETABLES		
Asparagus	6–7 stalks	20
Beans, green	½ cup	15
kidney	½ cup	335
lima	½ cup	80
Beets	½ cup	30
Broccoli	1 large stalk	30
Cabbage, raw	½ cup	12
cooked	½ cup	20
Carrots	1 medium or ½ cup	25
Cauliflower	½ cup	15
Celery	1 large stalk	5
Corn	5-inch ear or ½ cup	70
Cucumber	½ medium	5
Eggplant	2 slices or ½ cup	25
Green pepper	1	20
Lettuce	3 small leaves	3
Peas	½ cup	55
Potato, sweet	1 medium	200
white	1 medium	100
Potato chips	10	100
Radishes	2 small	4

APPENDIXES

Foods	Amount	Calories
Spinach	½ cup	25
Squash, summer	½ cup	15
winter	¼ cup	45
Tomato, raw	1 medium	30
canned or cooked	½ cup	25
FRUITS		
Apple	medium	75
Applesauce, unsweetened	½ cup	50
sweetened	½ cup	95
Apricots, raw	2 to 3	50
canned or dried	halves, 4 to 6	85
Avocado	½ small	250
Banana	medium	85
Cantaloupe	⅓ medium	35
Cherries, fresh	15 large	60
canned in syrup	½ cup	100
Cranberry sauce	½ cup	250
Fruit cocktail, canned	½ cup	90
Grapefruit	½ medium	55
Olive	1 large	8
Orange	1 medium	70
Peach, fresh	1 medium	45
canned in syrup	2 halves, 1 tbsp. juice	70
Pear, fresh	1 medium	45
canned in syrup	2 halves, 1 tbsp. juice	70
Pineapple, canned in syrup	1 slice	90
Plums, fresh	2 medium	50
canned in syrup	2 medium	75
Prunes, cooked with sugar	5 large	135
Raisins, dried	½ cup	200
Tangerine	1 large	45
CEREALS, BREADS, CRACKERS		
Puffed wheat	1 cup	45
Other dry cereal	average portion	100

Foods	Amount	Calories
Farina, cooked	¾ cup	100
Oatmeal, cooked	1 cup	135
Rice, cooked	1 cup	200
Macaroni or spaghetti, cooked	1 cup	200
Egg noodles, cooked	1 cup	100
Flour	1 cup	400
Bread, white, rye, or whole wheat	1 slice	70
Ry-Krisp	1 double square	20
Saltine	1 (2 inches square)	15
Ritz cracker	1	15
Biscuit	1 (2-inch diameter)	110
Hard roll	1 average	95
Pancakes	2 medium	130
Waffles	1 medium	230
Bun, cinnamon with raisins	1 average	185
Danish pastry	1 small	140
Muffin	1 medium	130

DAIRY PRODUCTS

Foods	Amount	Calories
Whole milk	1 cup	160
Evaporated milk	½ cup	170
Skim milk	1 cup	90
Buttermilk (from skim milk)	1 cup	90
Light cream, sweet or sour	1 tablespoon	30
Heavy cream	1 tablespoon	50
Yoghurt	1 cup	120
Whipped cream	1 tablespoon	50
Ice cream	⅙ quart	200
Cottage cheese	½ cup	100
Cheese	1 ounce or 1 slice	100
Butter	1 tablespoon	100
	1 pat	60
Egg, plain		80
fried or scrambled		110

DESSERTS

Foods	Amount	Calories
Chocolate layer cake	1/12 cake	350
Angel food cake	1/12 cake	115

APPENDIXES

Foods	Amount	Calories
Sponge cake	2 × 2¾ × ½ inches	100
Fruit pie	⅙ pie	375
Cream pie	⅙ pie	200
Lemon meringue pie	⅙ pie	280
Chocolate pudding	½ cup	220
Jell-O	1 serving	65
Fruit ice	½ cup	145
Doughnut, plain	1	130
Brownie	2 inches square	140
Cookie, plain	3-inch diameter	75

MISCELLANEOUS

Foods	Amount	Calories
Sugar, white	1 tablespoon (3 teaspoons)	50
Jam or jelly	1 tablespoon	60
Peanut butter	1 tablespoon	100
Catsup or chili sauce	2 tablespoons	35
White sauce, medium	¼ cup	100
Brown gravy	½ cup	80
Boiled dressing (cooked)	1 tablespoon	30
Mayonnaise	1 tablespoon	100
French dressing	1 tablespoon	60
Salad oil, olive oil, etc.	1 tablespoon	125
Margarine	1 tablespoon	100
Herbs and spices		0
Chocolate sauce	2 tablespoons	90
Cheese sauce	2 tablespoons	65
Butterscotch sauce	2 tablespoons	200

SNACKS

Foods	Amount	Calories
Chocolate bar	1 small	155
Chocolate creams	1 average size	50
Popcorn	1 cup popped	55
Potato chips	10 or ½ cup	100
Peanut or pistachio nut	1	5
Walnuts, pecans, filberts, or cashews	4 whole	40
Brazil nut	1	50
Butternut	1	25

Foods	Amount	Calories
Pickles	1 large sour	10
	1 average sweet	15
Chocolate nut sundae		270
BEVERAGES		
Chocolate milk	8-ounce glass	185
Cocoa made with milk	1 cup	175
Ice cream soda		255
Chocolate malted milk	1 glass	450
Eggnog (without liquor)	1 glass	235
Tea or coffee, plain		0
Apple juice or cider	½ cup	65
Grape juice	½ cup	90
Cola drink	8 ounces	95
Ginger ale	8 ounces	70
Grapefruit juice, unsweetened	½ cup	40
Pineapple juice	½ cup	55
Prune juice	½ cup	85
Tomato juice	½ cup	25
ALCOHOLIC BEVERAGES		
Beer	8 ounces	120
Wine	1 wine glass	75
Gin	1 jigger	115
Rum	1 jigger	125
Whiskey	1 jigger	120
Brandy	1 brandy glass	80
Cocktail	1 cocktail glass	150

APPENDIX E

The American Heart Association's Low-Fat, Low-Cholesterol Meal Plan

This plan is mainly for adults from their twenties on who have a family history of heart disease, or who may have increased their risks through a regular diet high in saturated fat and cholesterol. Children and adolescents, especially from susceptible families, can also benefit from this meal plan by forming tastes for food early in life that may protect them from heart disease when they reach adulthood.

The types of food recommended here are suitable for most people from childhood through maturity. The *amounts* of food specified in the food list, however, are recommended mainly for the average adult. Nutritional needs differ during growth periods of infants, children, and adolescents, and during pregnancy and breast feeding; at these times, the amounts of food to be eaten should be regulated by a physician.

To use this plan, simply select, every day, foods from each of the basic food groups in lists 1–5, and follow the recommendations for number and size of servings.

1. Meat, Poultry, Fish, Dried Beans and Peas, Nuts, Eggs

One serving: 3 to 4 ounces of cooked meat or fish (not including bone or fat) or 3 to 4 ounces of a vegetable listed here. Use two or more servings (a total of 6 to 8 ounces) daily.

RECOMMENDED	AVOID OR USE SPARINGLY
Chicken, turkey, veal, fish: Use in most of your meat meals for the week. Shellfish (clams, crab, lobster, oysters, scallops, shrimp) are low in fat but high in cholesterol. Use a 4-ounce serving as a substitute for meat no more than twice a week. *Beef, lamb, pork, ham:* Use in no more than five meals per week. Choose lean ground meat and lean cuts of meat; trim all visible fat before cooking; bake, broil, roast or stew so that you can discard the fat that cooks out of the meat. *Nuts and dried beans and peas.* Kidney beans, lima beans, baked beans, lentils, chick peas (garbanzos), and split peas are high in vegetable protein and may be used in place of meat occasionally. Egg whites may be used as desired.	Duck and goose. Heavily marbled and fatty meats, spare ribs, mutton, frankfurters, sausages, fatty hamburgers, bacon, luncheon meats. Organ meats (liver, kidney, heart, sweetbreads) are very high in cholesterol. Since liver is very rich in vitamins and iron, it should not be eliminated from the diet completely. Use a 4-ounce serving in a meat meal no more than once a week. Egg yolks: limit to 3 per week including eggs used in cooking. Cakes, batters, sauces, and other foods containing egg yolks.

2. Vegetables and Fruits (Fresh, frozen, or canned)

One serving: ½ cup. Use at least four servings daily.

RECOMMENDED	AVOID OR USE SPARINGLY
One serving should be a source of Vitamin C. Broccoli, cabbage (raw), tomatoes, berries, cantaloupes, grapefruits (or juice), mangoes,	Olives and avocados are very high in fat calories and should be used in moderation. If you must limit your calories, use vegetables such as potatoes,

APPENDIXES

RECOMMENDED
melons, oranges (or juice), papayas, strawberries, tangerines. *One serving should be a source of Vitamin A—dark green leafy or yellow vegetables, or yellow fruits.*
Broccoli, carrots, chard, chicory, escarole, greens (beet, collard, dandelion, mustard, turnip), kale, peas, rutabagas, spinach, string beans, sweet potatoes and yams, watercress, winter squash, yellow corn.
Apricots, cantaloupes, mangoes, papayas.
Other vegetables and fruits are also very nutritious; they should be eaten in salads, main dishes, snacks, and desserts, *in addition* to the recommended daily allowances of high vitamin A and C vegetables and fruits.

AVOID OR USE SPARINGLY
corn, or lima beans sparingly. To add variety to your diet, one serving (½ cup) of any one of these may be substituted for one serving of bread or cereals.

3. BREADS AND CEREALS (Whole grain, enriched, or restored)

One serving of bread: 1 slice. One serving of cereal: ½ cup, cooked; 1 cup, cold, with skimmed milk. Use at least four servings daily.

RECOMMENDED
Breads made with a minimum of saturated fat.
White enriched (including raisin bread), whole wheat, English muffins, French bread, Italian bread, oatmeal bread, pumpernickel, rye.
Biscuits, muffins, and griddle

AVOID OR USE SPARINGLY
Butter rolls; commercial biscuits, muffins, doughnuts, sweet rolls, cakes, crackers; egg bread, cheese bread; commercial mixes containing dried eggs and whole milk.

RECOMMENDED

cakes made at home, using an allowed liquid oil as shortening.

Cereals (hot and cold), rice, melba toast, matzos, pretzels.

Pasta: macaroni, noodles (except egg noodles), spaghetti.

4. Milk Products

One serving: 8 ounces (1 cup). Buy only skimmed milk that has been fortified with Vitamins A and D. Daily servings: Children up to twelve, 3 or more cups; Adults, 2 or more cups.

RECOMMENDED	AVOID OR USE SPARINGLY
Milk products that are low in dairy fats.	*Whole milk and whole milk products.*
Fortified skimmed (nonfat) milk and fortified skimmed milk powder, lof-fat milk. The label on the container should show that the milk is fortified with Vitamins A and D. The word "fortified" alone is not enough.	Chocolate milk; canned whole milk; ice cream; all creams including sour, half and half, whipped; whole milk yoghurt.
	Nondairy cream substitutes (usually coconut oil which is very high in saturated fat).
Buttermilk made from skimmed milk, yoghurt made from skimmed milk, canned evaporated skimmed milk, cocoa made with low-fat milk.	Cheeses made from cream or whole milk.
	Butter.
Cheeses made from skimmed or partially skimmed milk, such as cottage cheese, creamed or uncreamed (uncreamed, preferably); farmer's, baker's, or hoop cheese; mozzarella and sapsago cheeses made with partially skimmed milk.	

5. Fats and Oils (Polyunsaturated)

An individual allowance should include about 2 to 4 tablespoons daily (depending on how many calories you can afford) in the form of margarine, salad dressing, and shortening.

RECOMMENDED

Margarines, liquid oil shortenings, salad dressings, and mayonnaise containing any of these polyunsaturated vegetable oils.

Corn oil, cottonseed oil, safflower oil, sesame seed oil, soybean oil, sunflower seed oil.

Margarines and other products highly polyunsaturated usually can be identified by their label, which lists a recommended *liquid* vegetable oil as the *first* ingredient and one or more partially hydrogenated vegetable oils as additional ingredients.

Diet margarines are low in calories because they are low in fat. Therefore it takes twice as much diet margarine to supply the polyunsaturates contained in a recommended margarine.

AVOID OR USE SPARINGLY

Solid fats and shortenings.

Butter, lard, salt pork fat, meat fat, completely hydrogenated margarines and vegetable shortenings, products containing coconut oil.

Peanut oil and olive oil may be used occasionally for flavor, but they are low in polyunsaturates and do not take the place of the recommended oils.

6. Desserts, Beverages, Snacks, Condiments

The foods on this list are acceptable because they are low in saturated fat and cholesterol. If you have eaten your daily allowance from the first five lists, however, these foods will be in excess of your nutritional needs, and many of them may also exceed your calorie limits for maintaining a desirable weight. If you must limit your calories, limit your portions of the foods on this list as well.

Moderation should be observed, especially in the use of alcoholic drinks, ice milk, sherbet, sweets, and bottled drinks.

ACCEPTABLE

Low in calories or no calories.
Fresh fruit and fruit canned without sugar; tea, coffee (no cream), cocoa powder; water ices; gelatin; fruit whip; puddings made with nonfat milk; sweets and bottled drinks made with artificial sweeteners; vinegar, mustard, ketchup, herbs, spices.

High in calories.
Frozen or canned fruit with sugar added; jelly, jam, marmalade, honey; pure sugar candy such as gum drops, hard candy, mint patties (not chocolate); imitation ice cream made with safflower oil; cakes, pies, cookies, and puddings made with polyunsaturated fat in place of solid shortening; angel food cake; nuts, especially walnuts; nonhydrogenated peanut butter; bottled drinks, fruit drinks; ice milk; sherbet; wine, beer, whiskey.

AVOID OR USE SPARINGLY

Coconut and coconut oil; commercial cakes, pies, cookies, and mixes; frozen cream pies; commercially fried foods such as potato chips and other deep-fried snacks; whole milk puddings; chocolate pudding (high in cocoa butter and therefore high in saturated fat); ice cream.

APPENDIX F

Mild Sodium-restricted Diet: 1,800 Calories*

FOLLOW THIS DIET EVERY DAY

What to Have Each Day and How Much	Use	Things to Know	Do Not Use
MILK **2 glasses** *Each glass contains about 170 calories.*	Regular (whole) milk, evaporated milk, skim milk, buttermilk, reconstituted powdered milk. If you use skim milk, buttermilk, or powdered milk, you may add extra fat to your diet to make up for the fat that has been removed from the milk. For each glass, add 2 servings of fat. **Substitutes** for not more than 1 glass of milk a day: 2 ounces of meat, poultry, or fish or 6 ounces of plain yogurt (¾ cup).	A glass of milk = 1 cup (8 ounces). A half cup of evaporated milk counts as a glass of milk. With powdered milk, follow the directions on the box for making 1 cup.	Because of the extra calories they contain: ice cream, sherbet, malted milk, milk shakes, instant cocoa mixes, chocolate milk, condensed milk, and all other kinds of milk and fountain drinks.
MEAT, POULTRY, FISH **2 servings** *Each serving contains about 75 calories per ounce.*	Fresh, frozen, or canned meat or poultry: any kind except those listed in the last column. Fish or shellfish (fresh, frozen, or canned): any kind except those listed in the last column. **Substitutes** for 1 ounce of meat, poultry, or fish: 1 egg, ¼ cup lightly salted cottage cheese, 1 ounce natural American cheddar or Swiss cheese, or 2 tablespoons low-sodium dietetic peanut butter.	An average serving of meat, poultry, or fish is 3 ounces. (Allow an extra ounce or two for shrinkage, bone, and fat when you shop.) Examples of 3-ounce servings: 1 pork chop; 2 rib lamb chops; half breast or leg and thigh of 3-pound chicken; 2 meat patties, 2 inches across and ½ inch thick; 2 thin slices roast meat, each 3 × 3 × ¼ inches.	Salty or smoked meat (bacon, bologna, chipped or corned beef, frankfurters, ham, meats koshered by salting, luncheon meats, salt pork, sausage, smoked tongue). Salty or smoked fish (anchovies, caviar, salted cod, herring, sardines, etc.). Processed cheese or cheese spreads unless low-sodium dietetic; cheese such as Roquefort, Camembert, or Gorgonzola. Regular peanut butter.
VEGETABLES **At least 3 servings** *Each starchy vegetable serving contains about 70 calories.* *Other vegetables contain from 5 to 35 calories per serving.*	Any fresh, frozen, or canned vegetables or vegetable juices, except those listed in the last column.	Count as a serving: about ½ cup.	Sauerkraut, pickles, or other vegetables prepared in brine or heavily salted.
FRUIT **4 servings** *Each serving contains about 40 calories.*	Any kind of fruit or fruit juice—fresh, frozen, canned, or dried—if sugar has not already been added.	The size of a serving of fruit varies, depending on the fruit and the calories. Examples: 1 small apple, ½ cup fruit cup, 2 medium plums, 1 cup strawberries, 1 cup watermelon.	Because of the extra calories they contain: fruits canned or frozen in sugar syrup.

BREADS, CEREALS, AND CEREAL PRODUCTS **7 servings** *Each serving contains about 70 calories.*	Breads, rolls, and lightly salted crackers; lightly salted cooked cereals; dry cereals; matzos; melba toast; macaroni, noodles, spaghetti, rice, barley; lightly salted popcorn; flour. **Substitute** for a serving of bread or cereal: a starchy vegetable.	Count as a serving: 1 slice bread, 1 roll or muffin, 4 crackers or pieces of melba toast, ½ cup cooked cereal, ¾ cup dry cereal, ½ cup cooked noodles or rice, etc., 1½ cups popcorn, 2½ tablespoons flour.	Breads and rolls with salt topping; regular salted popcorn, potato chips, corn chips, pretzels, etc. *Because of the extra calories they contain:* sugar-coated cereals, pastries, cakes, sweet rolls, and cookies.
FAT **4 servings** *Each serving contains about 45 calories.*	Butter or margarine, cooking fat or oil, French dressing, mayonnaise, heavy or light cream, unsalted nuts, avocado.	Count as a serving: 1 level teaspoon (or small pat) butter, margarine, fat, oil, or mayonnaise; 1 tablespoon heavy cream (sweet or sour); 2 tablespoons light cream; 1 tablespoon French dressing; 6 small nuts; ⅛ of 4-inch avocado.	Bacon and bacon fat, salt pork, olives, salted nuts, and party spreads and dips and other heavily salted snack foods, such as potato chips and sticks, crackers, etc.
AND...TAKE YOUR CHOICE **Choose 2** *Each choice contains about 75 calories.*	Each of these is one choice: Two servings of fruit; one serving of bread, cereal, or starchy vegetable; two servings of fat; four teaspoons of sugar, honey, syrup, molasses, jelly, jam, or marmalade; candy made without salted nuts (75 calories' worth).	These choices are intended to give you more freedom in planning your day's meals. They are part of your diet, and you are to include them every day. You may split these choices if you wish. For example, one serving of fruit and 2 teaspoons of sugar could make 1 choice.	If you do want sweetened fruit or juice, add an allowed sugar substitute or the amount of sugar, honey, etc., allowed on the list headed And...Take Your Choice.
MISCELLANEOUS	As desired: coffee, tea, coffee substitutes, unsweetened or low-calorie soft drinks; sugar substitutes; lemons, limes; gelatin; vinegar; cream of tartar; baking powder, baking soda (for baking only); yeast.	If your calories are not restricted, see additional foods allowed under Changes for Unrestricted Calories.	Canned soups, stews; any kind of commercial bouillon—cubes, powders, or liquids. *Because of the extra calories they contain:* baking chocolate; cocoa and cocoa mixes; fruit-flavored beverage mixes; sugar-sweetened soft drinks, custards, gelatin desserts, puddings; cornstarch, cornmeal, and tapioca.

USE ONLY HALF THE SALT AND MONOSODIUM GLUTAMATE YOU USED TO USE.

*If your doctor wants you to have only 1,200 calories, or if he says you do not need to restrict your calories, make the appropriate changes described below.

Changes for 1,200 Calories
MILK: Use skim milk, buttermilk, or powdered milk only, and do not add the extra fat. You may substitute 1 ounce of meat, poultry, or fish for 1 glass of milk a day. BREADS, ETC.: 4 servings instead of 7. FAT: No servings instead of 4. AND... TAKE YOUR CHOICE: 1 choice instead of 2. (Note: You can have fat as a "choice" even though the other 4 servings of fat are omitted.)

Changes for Unrestricted Calories
EXTRA SERVINGS: You may have extra servings of any allowed food.
ADDITIONAL FOODS: You may have any of the foods that are ruled out above *because of the calories.* You may also have alcoholic beverages (with your doctor's permission).

APPENDIX G

If You Want to Give Up Cigarettes

(Excerpted from the American Cancer Society booklet of the same title, reproduced here with the Society's permission)

ONCE YOU HAVE STOPPED

If you are like most cigarette smokers, you will in two weeks or less say farewell to that hacking, shattering morning cough, good-bye to ugly thick phlegm, adios to smoker's headaches and unpleasant cigarette-induced mouth and stomach complaints.

You will be saving—how much? Well, how much do you smoke up in dollars every week? Could be considerable.

You will no longer burn cigarette holes in clothing, furniture, rugs, or tablecloths. Food will tend to taste better and your sense of smell will return to normal. Cigarette breath (it can be very offensive) will disappear.

Q Day, cigarette quitting day, might well be renamed K Day—kindness day for both you and your friends. By quitting cigarettes you are instituting an immediate program of kindness to your lungs, your heart, your stomach, your nose, your throat.

A GARLAND OF FACTS

Since you have decided to give up cigarette smoking, you probably know the risks of the habit. However, a brief selection from the mountains of facts that have developed through research, published since 1954, may be useful.

Cigarette smoking used to be compared to Russian roulette. Now we know better. Every regular cigarette smoker is injured, though not in the same degree. Cigarette smoking kills some, makes others lung cripples, gives still others far more than their share of illness and loss of work days. Cigarette smoking is not a gamble; regular cigarette smokers studied at autopsy all show the effects.

The regular cigarette smoker runs a risk of death from lung cancer ten times greater than the nonsmoker; men who smoke more than a pack a day have about twenty times as much lung cancer as nonsmokers have. Unfortunately, early diagnosis of lung cancer is very difficult; only about one in twenty cases is cured.

Men aged twenty-five who have never smoked regularly can expect six and a half years more of life than men who smoke one pack or more a day. Twice as many heavy smokers (two packs a day) as nonsmokers will die between twenty-five and sixty-five years of age.

The average heavy smoker (two or more packs a day) smokes about three quarters of a million cigarettes during his lifetime. As a result, he loses about 4.4 million minutes—8.3 years—of life compared with nonsmokers. This amounts to a loss of almost six minutes per cigarette smoked; a minute of life for a minute of smoking.

Male smokers (ten or more cigarettes a day) between forty-five and fifty-four have more than three times the death rate from heart attacks than nonsmokers do. In the ages between forty and sixty-four, heart attacks prematurely kill some 45,000 cigarette-smoking men.

Cigarette smokers between forty-five and sixty-four miss 50 percent more days at work than do nonsmokers. Or, to say it another way: According to the Public Health Service, if cigarette smokers had the same rate of illness as nonsmokers, some 77 million working days would not be lost annually.

Emphysema, a relatively rare disease a few years ago, is now a major cause of medical disability in this country. Most emphysema is caused by cigarette smoking. The disease is both a crippler and a killer, causing the lungs to lose their elasticity. Eventually the effort to breathe becomes a constant, agonizing struggle.

A longer and healthier life is high on our priorities: giving up cigarette smoking is the most important action that the average individual can take that will improve the physical quality of his daily life, extend his life expectancy, and increase his chances of avoiding lung cancer, heart disease, emphysema, and a number of other nasty complaints.

As You Approach Q Day

Many stress willpower as the decisive factor in giving up cigarettes. For them the sense that they can manage their own lives is of great importance. They enjoy challenging themselves and, with an effort of will, they break the cigarette habit.

Thus, some psychologists describe stopping cigarettes as an exercise in self-mastery, one that introduces a new dimension of self-control.

Others, often successful in many aspects of living, find that willpower does not help them in giving up cigarettes. They try to stop, they do not, and they feel guilty over their weakness. This is a mistake, since many smokers fail in their first and second, even their fifth attempts, and then finally succeed. Those whose "will" fails in breaking the habit are not weak but different. Their approach must be less through determination and more through relearning new behavior with patience and perseverance.

Self-suggestion, when one is relaxed, aimed at changing one's feelings and thoughts about cigarettes can be useful.

One health educator remarked recently, "Nothing succeeds like willpower and a little blood in the sputum."

To think of stopping smoking as self-denial is an error; the ex-smoker should not believe that he is giving up an object of value, however dependent he may be on it. If he begins to feel sorry for himself and broods on his sufferings, they may well become more severe and indeed unendurable. He must recognize that he is teaching himself a more positive, more constructive, more rewarding behavior.

Try Cutting Down

An important first step in the process of giving up cigarettes for many smokers is to set the date for Q Day, when you are going to stop completely, and, as it approaches, to gradually reduce the number of cigarettes you smoke, day by day or week by week.

A good system is to decide to smoke only once an hour—or to stop smoking between the hours of 9 and 10 o'clock, 11 and 12, 1 and 2, 3 and 4, etc. And then to extend the nonsmoking time by half an hour, an hour, two hours.

You may decide to halve the cigarettes you smoke week by week, giving yourself four weeks to Q Day.

How about smoking only half of each cigarette?

In the process of reducing the number of daily cigarettes, try various possibilities: if you have one pocket in which you always carry your pack, put it in another so that you will have to fumble for it. If you always use your right hand to bring your cigarette to your mouth, use the left hand. Is it your custom to rest the cigarette in the right corner of the mouth? Try the left side.

Make it a real effort to get a cigarette. Wrap your package in several sheets of paper or place it in a tightly covered box. If you leave your change at home you won't be able to use a cigarette machine.

Shift from cigarettes you like to an unpalatable brand.

Before you light up, ask yourself, "Do I really want this cigarette or am I just acting out of empty habit?"

A smoker may find an unlighted cigarette in the mouth is helpful. Others enjoy handling and playing with a cigarette.

Cigarette smoking is a habit that is usually very well learned—learning the habit of not smoking can be difficult. It can help in breaking into your habit chain to make yourself aware of the nature and frequency of your smoking behavior.

Score Card

Many smokers have found that a useful step in understanding their smoking is the keeping of a daily record on a scale like this:

NEED	MORNING HOURS (A.M.)							AFTERNOON						EVENING HOURS (P.M.)					
	6	7	8	9	10	11	12	1	2	3	4	5	6	7	8	9	10	11	12	1
1																				
2																				
3																				
4																				
5																				
6																				

Copy this record sheet seven times for seven days. Make a check for each cigarette you smoke, hour by hour, and indicate how much you need it: a mark in the box opposite 1 shows low need, a mark opposite 6, high need; opposite 4, moderate need, etc. Then decide which cigarette you wish to eliminate.

In your gradual withdrawal you may decide to eliminate those daily cigarettes that you find are rated 1, 2, or 3, i.e., ones you want least. Or you may wish to give up first the cigarettes you like most. In any case keeping a smoking log will give you information about yourself and make you more aware of what your smoking habits are.

You may find that you are largely a social smoker, that smoking makes you feel closer to others, more welcome at a party; that you seem to have more friends. A cigarette may play a surprisingly large part in your picture of yourself as a mature and successful person.

How do you convince yourself that people like and respect you for more important reasons than for your cigarette? Try not smoking and see.

PLUS AND MINUS

Write down carefully, after some thought, in one column the reasons why you smoke and in another all the reasons why you should give up cigarettes.

As you turn this exercise over in your mind, new material will occur to you for one or the other columns. Thoughtful concentration on your reasons for giving up cigarettes is important in changing your behavior.

Four Smoking Styles

Dr. Silvan Tomkins distinguishes four general types of smoking behavior. An abbreviated summary of the types follows:

Habitual smoking. Here the smoker may hardly be aware that he has a cigarette in his mouth. He smokes as if it made him feel good, or feel better, but in fact it does neither. He may once have regarded smoking as an important sign of status. But now smoking is automatic. The habitual smoker who wants to give up must first become aware of when he is smoking. Knowledge of the pattern of his smoking is a first step toward change.

Positive-affect smoking. Here smoking is used as a stimulant that produces exciting pleasure or as a relaxant to heighten enjoyment, as at the end of a meal. Here a youngster demonstrates his manhood or his defiance of his parents. This smoker may enjoy most the handling of a cigarette or the sense and sight of smoke curling out of his mouth. If these smokers can be persuaded to make an effort, they may find giving up cigarettes relatively painless.

Negative-affect smoking. This is sedative smoking, using the habit to reduce feelings of distress, fear, shame, or disgust or any combination of them. This person may not smoke at all when things go well, on vacation or at a party, but under tension, when things go badly at the office or at home, he reaches for a cigarette. These smokers give up often, but when the heat and pressure of the day hit them, when there's a challenge, they find it very hard to resist a cigarette. A strong substitute, like nibbling ginger root, may be useful.

Addictive smoking. The smoker is always aware when he is not smoking. The absence of a cigarette is uncomfortably obvious. The lack of a cigarette builds need, desire, and discomfort at not smoking. With this increasing need is the expectation that a cigarette will reduce discomfort—and the cigarette does give relief—for a moment. Pleasure at smoking is real, just as the buildup of discomfort at not smoking is real, sometimes rapid and intolerable. The enjoyment of the cigarette, however, is very brief, and may be disappointing—but the suffering for lack of slight relief is considerable. For this smoker, tapering off doesn't seem to work: the only solution is to quit cold. Once you have been through the intense pain of breaking your psychological addiction, you are unlikely to start smoking again. The experience of giving up has been too uncomfortable—and too memorable for you to risk having to go through it again.

Some such smokers have found it useful to increase during the week before Q Day the number of cigarettes smoked, to go from two packs to four packs, to force themselves to smoke so that their bodies will be in actual revolt against the double dose of tar and nicotine.

For information on a Smoker's Self-Testing Kit (four questionnaires, etc., to help one to understand personal reasons for, and style of, smoking) write to the National Clearinghouse for Smoking and Health, United States Public Health Service, 40404 North Fairfax Drive, Arlington, Va. 22203.

The Week Before Q Day

Think over your list of reasons why you should not smoke: the risk of disease, the blurring of the taste of food, the cost, the cough, the bad breath, the mess and smell of morning-after ashtrays.

Concentrate each evening when you are relaxed, just before you fall asleep, on one result of cigarette smoking. Repeat and repeat and repeat that single fact. Drive home another fact the next night and another the next.

Review the facts that you know about the risks of cigarette smoking. Remind yourself that there, but for the grace of God, go you; that you may indeed, if you continue smoking, lose six and a half years of life; that—if you are a heavy smoker—your chances of dying between twenty-five and sixty-five years of age are twice as great as those of the nonsmoker. Are the six minutes of pleasure in a cigarette worth six minutes fewer of life to a heavy smoker? Would you fly in an airplane if the chances of crash and death were even close to the risks of cigarette smoking? Think over why it is that 100,000 physicians have quit cigarette smoking.

APPENDIXES

ACTION: Q DAY

Let us suppose that you know, now, when and where and how you smoke. You have suggested again and again to your tired mind that smoking is a dangerous business.

"But what will I do the morning of Q Day when, mind or no mind, I desperately want a cigarette?"

We hope you will prove that you are stronger than your dependence. Here are some tips that may prove useful when you have an impulse to smoke. They are not scientifically proven, but many smokers have found one or another of them helpful.

For the mouth. Drink frequent glasses of water.

Nibble fruit, cookies, eat somewhat self-pleasing food.

Suck candy mints and/or chew gum (sugarless gum will be easier on your teeth).

Chew bits of fresh ginger when you start to reach for a cigarette. (Take this gently; ginger root is aromatic and pervasive—some experience it as burning, others as clean and satisfying.)

Bite a clove.

Nicotine replacement. Lobeline sulphate tablets, available without prescription, are reported to make it easier for some people to stop cigarettes. Authorities disagree as to whether they provide a substitute that will help satisfy your body's craving for nicotine.

(Since some individuals—those with stomach ulcers, for instance—should not use these tablets, check with your physician before trying them.)

Be vigorous: exercise. Strenuous physical activity that demands effort and keeps you busy can be very helpful.

Vacation is a good time for some people to stop: camping, mountain climbing, tennis.

Stretching exercises or long walks can be relaxing.

Go "no smoking." For a few days, spend as much time as possible in libraries or other places where smoking is forbidden. Ride in "No Smoking" cars.

A spurt of motion picture or theater-going will pass many hours.

Keep away for two weeks from friends who are heavy smokers.

Use your lungs. Deep breaths of air can be wonderfully calming.

Inhalers—that reduce nasal stuffiness—may help tide you over the first few days.

After meals. For some the cigarette after breakfast coffee or at the end of lunch or dinner is most important. Instead of a cigarette try a mouth wash after each meal.

If you have had a specific pattern that you have followed after dinner you may want to change it: read a book instead of a newspaper, skip familiar television programs, sit in another comfortable chair, try crossword puzzles, take care of some household task you have been putting off, take your dog out for a walk.

On the other hand, you may prefer to do all the things that are familiar and comfortable for you and to which you are used—except to smoke cigarettes. Take your choice.

Reward yourself. Be sure you have your favorite food on Q Day.

Give yourself all the things that you like best—except cigarettes.

When you have saved a bit of money by not smoking, buy yourself a present: perhaps a new record, or a blouse, or necktie, or book, or a trinket.

So—Now You Are on Your Own

When the impulse to smoke is strong, try a substitute: a drink of water, a piece of gum, a walk around the block, stretching, and deep breathing.

These substitutes may only satisfy you temporarily—but they will keep you alert and aware and will soften the strength of your desire to smoke. Equally important are constant reminders to yourself of why you are stopping cigarettes. Remember the reasons that you put down for not smoking. Recall the basic data about disease, disability, and death that are caused by cigarettes.

You may be very uncomfortable, but "this too shall pass" relates to cigarette-less shakes, irritation and temper, the urge to climb walls, depression, anxiety. Time is a great healer.

A minority of cigarette smokers go through the terrors of the damned after they quit. Even these—when they come on the fresh air side—report great pride at having been able to give up.

Unfortunately, fear of failure to make it seems to deter very many men and women from even trying—but for many, giving up cigarettes, while uncomfortable and a strain, is by no means agony. After all their terrible expectations, stopping can seem relatively easy.

Questions and Answers

Do you believe in cold turkey quitting? Yes for some, no for others. If you are a really "addicted" smoker, psychologists favor the sudden, decisive break. For some, gradual withdrawal is less painful and entirely satisfactory.

Some cigarette smokers shift to pipes and cigars—there is of course some risk of mouth cancer from these but overall mortality of cigar and pipe smokers is only a little higher than among nonsmokers, provided the smoke is not inhaled.

What about going to a cigarette withdrawal clinic for help? If there is a clinic or program in your community, you may find it useful. The American Cancer Society favors such efforts. Sharing your withdrawal experiences with others and working with them on a common problem can be very helpful. The clinic may make it considerably easier in various ways to stop cigarette smoking. However, remember, no clinic can provide a sure result. In this matter you must be both patient and physician.

Shall I make a big thing of Q Day? Some find it most satisfactory to work on a schedule in which Q Day, quitting day, is singled out as the important, decisive day in their personal lives—which indeed it is.

Others who have known for a long time that cigarettes are bad for them and that sooner or later they will stop, wake up one morning and say to themselves, "This is it. No more cigarettes."

What motivates them? An obituary, an antismoking commercial on television, a magazine article, a leaflet brought home from school by a child, a worried look from their son, being fed up with a repeated cough. There are many possible stimuli to stop, but almost always beneath the casual-seeming but bold decision are months, often years, of thought and worry.

What if I fail to make it? Don't be discouraged; many thousands who stopped did so only after several attempts.

Some people prefer to stop for just one day at a time. They promise themselves twenty-four hours of freedom from cigarettes, and when the day is over they make a commitment to themselves for one more day. And another. And another. At the end of any twenty-four-hour period they can go back to cigarettes without betraying themselves—but they usually do not.

Is smoking a real addiction? This depends on your definition of words. In any case, smokers obviously can become very strongly, very tragically dependent on cigarettes.

However, the discomfort that most feel at giving up cigarettes is not like the painful withdrawal symptoms that drug addicts report.

Giving up cigarettes is much closer to the discomfort and the irritation produced by dieting than to the agony of stopping drugs. As so many know, dieting in an effort to lose fifteen or twenty pounds can be a most uncomfortable experience—but when you have done it, you have a fine feeling.

Shall I throw out our ashtrays? One school of thought asks, Do you leave a bottle of whiskey near an alcoholic? Their recommendation is to get rid of cigarettes, ashtrays, anything that might remind a smoker of his former habit.

Others take a different view and even suggest carrying cigarettes to demonstrate to yourself that you can resist temptation. Choose for yourself.

Shall I tell others of my decision? Some do, some don't. Some find that the wider they spread the news of their decision the easier it is for them to make it stick. Others regard not smoking as their own personal business and keep it almost entirely to themselves. Will you strengthen your decision if your wife and friends know that you have committed yourself?

Will I gain weight? Many do. Food is a substitute for cigarettes for many people. And your appetite may be fresher and stronger.

During the first few weeks of giving up cigarettes some psychologists recommend pampering yourself: eating well, drinking well, enjoying those things that are pleasant and fulfilling.

Some people, those to whom self-mastery is vital, get rewards out of controlling their wish for fattening food at the same time that they are licking the urge for cigarettes. Again, it depends upon the person and his approach.

How about hypnosis? There is much interest in this technique by some physicians who report success, particularly with hard-core smokers. Why not discuss the matter with a physician, if you are interested.

Shall I see my physician? Yes. However, the problem is yours, not his, and he may not feel that he can be helpful. On the other hand he may be able to give you sympathetic support and may prescribe medication. He can be helpful, also, in suggesting a diet that will prevent you from gaining too much weight.

Physicians as a profession have been leaders in acting on the risks of cigarette smoking: the Public Health Service estimates that 100,000 physicians (half the physicians who once were cigarette smokers) have kicked the habit. A California study shows that only 21.3 percent of all physicians in the state are cigarette smokers now.

Why do so many people smoke cigarettes? Surely one reason is that the cigarette industry spends about $300 million a year in promoting the habit and in challenging the facts that scientists have produced that point to the dangers of the habit.

Another reason is that something in cigarettes, probably nicotine, is habit-forming; smokers become dependent rather rapidly on cigarettes.

Cigarette smoking is essentially a twentieth-century habit, encouraged by wars, by brilliant advertising, and by the development of remarkably efficient automatic machinery that produces those millions of round firmly packed cigarettes.

It is only within the last fifteen years that we have learned, through research pioneered by the American Cancer Society, that this personal and socially accepted habit is extremely dangerous. Cigarette smoking is deeply embedded in our life: agriculture, industry, government, the communications media all have a stake in it. It is still widely accepted, even though proven to be a most certain hazard to health.

Because promotion is important in maintaining the habit's popularity, the Society believes all cigarette advertising in all media should be terminated. We hope that this goal will be achieved voluntarily and that governmental action won't be necessary.

Index

Activities: after heart attack, 60-70; calorie expenditure and, 107-8, 227; dynamic, 68; isometric, 68-69; social, 76; to be avoided, 67-69; weight reduction and, 104; *see also* Exercise
Adrenal glands, 211; hormones, 26, 96, 110; response to stress, 110, 123; tumor, 88
Age, *see* Old age
Aggression, 115
Airplanes, travel in, 73
Air swallowing (aerophagia), 17
Alcoholic beverages, 75-76
Alcoholic myocardiopathy, 75
Allopurinol, 131
American Cancer Society, 122, 253, 255; booklet on smoking, 244-56
American Diabetes Association, 134
American Heart Association, 79, 189, 190, 200; diet plan, 99, 105, 200-201, 235-40
American Lung Association, 119
Angina (angina pectoris), 22-32, 81, 211; abdominal, 31; after heart attack, 59-62; atherosclerosis and, 27-28, 31-32; cardiospasm confused with, 16; chest pains confused with, 16-17, 31, 32; coronary bypass and, 177-78, 184; description of, 22-24; diagnosis of, 31-32; exercise and, 62, 67, 69, 118; nitroglycerin for, 32, 67, 157-61, *see also* Nitroglycerin; pain of heart attack compared with, 32, 34; propranolol for, 162-64; sexual activity and, 71; smoking and, 78; work and, 66-67, 69
Anticoagulants, 167-72, 211; aspirin and other drugs with, 169-70; in heart attack, 170-72

Anxiety, 211; with heart attack, 34, 55-58
Aorta, 25, 26, 88, 197, 212; in bypass surgery, 182; coarctation of, 140
Arrhythmia, 212; *see also* Heart rhythm
Arteries, 212; atherosclerosis in, other than coronary, 30-31; coronary, *see* Coronary arteries; femoral, 202; mammary, 181; pulmonary, 25; surgery for, 31, *see also* Coronary bypass
Arteriosclerosis, *see* Atherosclerosis
Arthritis, 16-17
Artificial heart, 205-6
Artificial respiration, 190-91, 193
Aspirin, 61, 172-73; anticoagulants and, 169-70; products containing, 169-70; reactions to, 151, 152
Atherosclerosis, 26-31, 212, 214; age related to, 29; angina and, 27-28, 31-32; blood fat levels and, 201-2; exercise and, 107; heart attack and, 37-38, 50; hypertension and, 87-88; lipids in blood and, 94-96; smoking and, 202; surgery for, 31; in women, 30
Atrial fibrillation, 75
Auricles (atria), 25, 197, 212
Auscultation, 142, 212
Automobiles: driving, 72; riding in, 72-73

Balloon, intra-aortic, 46, 53
Bathing after heart attack, 63
Beck, Claude, 181
Bendroflumethiazide, 155
Benzthiazide, 155
Beta blockers, 161
Bicycling, 68, 117
Biofeedback in hypertension, 92

257

Birth control pills, 30, 71, 78, 88; as risk factors, 82, 84-85; smoking and, 120
Blood: circulation of, 24-26; clotting and anticoagulants, 167-72; enzymes in, 42; fats in, 77, 83, 93, 201-4, 213, see also Cholesterol, Lipids, Triglycerides; glucose (sugar) in, 133-34, 136, 157; in healing after heart attack, 50-51; in heart attack, 38; nicotine harmful to, 77; tests, 148-49, 168; uric acid in, 130-31, 157
Blood clots in veins (phlebitis), 72-73, 85, 171
Blood pressure, 87, 213; high, see Hypertension; tests, 140
Boston: hyaluronidase studies, 204-5; Joslin Clinic, 132
Brain: arteries in, 30, see also Stroke; damage from fibrillation, 44
Breath, shortness of: exercise and, 69-70; in heart attack, 35
Bronchitis, chronic, 119
Buerger's disease, 119
Bursitis, 16

Cadmium in drinking water, 135
Caffeine, 155
Calories: energy expenditure of, 107-8, 227; in foods and beverages, 229-34; in reducing diet, 103-5
Cancer, lung, 77, 119
Car, see Automobiles
Carbohydrates, 133, 136-37
Cardiac arrest, 40, 193
Cardiac compression, 190-93
Cardiac neurosis, 20
Cardiopulmonary resuscitation (CPR), 189-93
Cardiospasm, 16
Catecholamines, 38, 77
Catheterization of heart and coronary artery, 147-48, 182, 213-14
Cervical root syndrome, 16-17
Charleston, W. Va., Physical Fitness for Senior Citizens, 113-14
Chest pain: after heart attack, 60-61; angina, 22-32, 34, see also Angina; birth control pills and, 85; causes other than heart disease, 15-21; exercise and, 63, 69-70; in heart attack, 34, 38, 46, 189
Children: diet for, 195-96; heart disease in, 195-96
Chlorothiazide, 155

Chlorthalidone, 155
Cholesterol: in body, 95-96; in children, 195-96; in diet, 78-79, 97-99, 195-96, 201, 203, 228; exercise and, 108-9; levels in blood, 96-98, 108-9, 127-28, 132, 201-3; as risk factor, 83, 84, 86, 93-101, 203; in stress, 127-28
Chromium deficiency in food, 136-37
Churchill, Winston, 69
Cigarettes, see Smoking
Claudication, 30, 214
Clofibrate, 101
Coarctation of aorta, 140, 214
Colchicine, 131
Collateral circulation, 28, 111-12, 214
Congenital heart defects, 186
Congestive heart failure, 53-54, 139-40, 152, 214
Contraceptives, oral, see Birth control pills
Coronary arteries, 26, 202, 214; catheterization, 147-48, 182; hypertension in, 88; obstruction of, 51
Coronary artery disease, see Atherosclerosis
Coronary bypass (coronary revascularization), 177-86; procedure, 181-83
Coronary care unit (CCU), 42-49
Coronary circulation, 26, 51, 111-12
Coronary Drug Project, 101
Coronary heart disease, see Heart disease
Coronary insufficiency, 69
Coronary occlusion, 214; see also Heart attack
Coronary thrombosis, 199, 214; see also Heart attack
Corticosteroids, 96
Cortisone, 61
Coumadin, 167-68

Dancing, 76
Death: attitude toward, 54, 55, 129-30, 138; sudden, and sedentary life, 112
Defibrillator, 45, 214
Depression: after heart attack, 56-58, 188; chest pain and, 19-20
Dextrothyroxine, 101
Diabetes (diabetes mellitus), 28, 136, 157; as risk factor, 83, 84, 132-34; symptoms, 132-33
Diaphragmatic hernia, 16
Dicumarol, 167-68
Diet: American Heart Association plan,

INDEX

99, 105, 200-201; calories in foods and beverages, 229-34; changes in, 78-79, 201-2; for children, 195-96; cholesterol in, *see* Cholesterol; in hospital after heart attack, 47-48; for hypertension, 89, 91-92; reducing, 103-5; salt- (sodium-) restricted, 78-79, 91-92, 197, 198, 204, 242-43

Digitalis, 53, 71, 152-55, 215; diuretics taken with, 153, 154, 156, 157; for heart failure, 197, 198; potassium deficiency and, 91; symptoms of overdose, 154-55

Digitoxin, 153

Digoxin, 153

Disopyramide (Norpace), 167

Diuretics, 53, 54, 71, 155-57, 215; digitalis taken with, 153, 154, 156, 157; for heart failure, 197; for hypertension, 89, 91, 92; side effects of, 156-57

Dressler's syndrome, 61

Drinking, 75-76

Drugs (medication), 150-74; anticoagulants, 167-72; for hypertension, 89-93, 162; for lipid levels in blood, 100-101; for pain relief, 46; for sedation, 47; side effects of, 90-91, 151-52, 156-57, 159, 163-69; weight-reducing, 103; *see also* names of drugs, as Aspirin, Nitroglycerin

Echocardiography, 146, 215

Eisenhower, Dwight D., 80, 188

Electrical heart failure, 36, 40-41

Electrocardiogram (ECG or EKG), 31, 39, 142-44, 215; in heart attack, 41; Holter, 144, 215; in stress test, 145

Emotional reactions: after heart attack, 47, 54-58; catecholamines and, 38; chest pain and, 19-20; in sports, 69

Emphysema, 119, 245-46

Energy: METS in measurement of, 65; required for work, 65-66

Enzymes, 216; in blood, 42

Estrogen, 101

Ethacrynic acid, 155

Examination, physical, 139-42

Exercise, 106-19; after meals, 64, 68, 69; blood lipid levels and, 108-9; dangers of, 69-70, 116; heart response to, 110-12; hypertension, 109; in old age, 113-16; program for, 116-19; in recovery from heart attack, 48-49, 60-65; in side effects of drugs, 91; sleep and, 112-13; in tension and stress, 109-10; for weight reduction, 107-8

Eyes, examination of, 141

Family: in inheritance of heart disease, 83-84; responsibility in heart attack, 187-89

Fatigue, 49, 60

Fats: in blood, 77, 83, 93, 201-4, *see also* Cholesterol, Lipids, Triglycerides; in diet, 78-79, 97-98, 200, 204; polyunsaturated and monounsaturated, 98; saturated, 97-98

Femoral artery, 202

Fever after heart attack, 50, 61

Fibrillation, 143, 216; atrial, 75; ventricular, 40, 43-45

Food, *see* Diet

Food poisoning, 17

Framingham Study, 85-86, 88, 94, 101, 112, 120, 130-32, 203, 204

Gallbladder disease, 15

Gitaligin, 153

Glossary, 211-25

Glucose: in blood, 133-34, 136, 157; in diabetes, 133, 134

Gout, 216; uric acid and, 130-31, 157

Heart: artificial, 205-6; of athletes, 110-11; catheterization of, 147-48, 182; description of, 24-26; exercise beneficial to, 110-12; recovery from attacks, 39-40, 50-52; smoking harmful to, 77; surgery, *see* Coronary bypass; tests and examinations, 139-49; transplants, 206-8

Heart attack, 33-58; after surgery, 184, 185; anticoagulants in, 170-72; atherosclerosis and, 37-38, 50; complications after, 52-54; emotional problems, *see* Emotional reactions; family of patient, 187-89; first aid (resuscitation), 189-93; healing after, 39-40, 50-52; heart failure distinguished from, 196-97; hospital care in, 41-49, 52; inheritance as factor in, 83-84; life after, 59-80; medical help in emergency, 35-37, 41-42; nationality, race, and sex as factors in, 82; pain in, 34, 38, 46; pain of angina compared with, 32, 34; personality related to, 125-30; pump failure in, 204-5; recovery after, 39-40, 50-52; repeated, 54-55, 79-81; risk factors, 83-

Heart attack (*continued*)
138; severity of, 38-39; silent (mild), 33-34; survival rate of patients, 43; symptoms of, 34-35, 38
Heartbeat, 25-26, 40; apex beat, 141; pulse and, 139; *see also* Heart rhythm
Heartburn, 16
Heart disease: in children, prevention of, 195-96; congenital defects, 195; mortality from, 199-201
Heart failure: congestive, mild, 53-54, 139-40, 152; electrical, 36, 40-41; heart attack distinguished from, 196-97; sudden death, 35-36; treatment of, 197-98
Heart-lung machine, 183, 205, 217
Heart murmurs, 142
Heart rhythm: alcohol as influence on, 75; digitalis and, 152; disturbances in exercise, 69-70, 118; drugs affecting, 161-67; fibrillation, *see* Fibrillation; hyaluronidase treatment for, 204-5; monitoring in heart attack, 42; treatment of abnormalities, 43-45; ventricular tachycardia, 40
Heberden, William, 22
Heparin, 167-68, 217
Heredity, *see* Inheritance
Hernia, hiatus (diaphragmatic), 16
Herrick, J. B., 199
Holter ECG, 144, 215
Hospital: coronary care unit (CCU), 42-49; emergency care in, 41-42; postcoronary care in, 49, 52, 60
Household work, 67-69
Hyaluronidase, 204-5
Hydrochlorothiazide, 155
Hydroflumethiazide, 155
Hyperlipemia, 96, 217
Hypertension (high blood pressure), 28, 83-93, 139; biofeedback in, 92; blood fat levels and, 201-2; causes of, 88-89; dangers of, 87; in diabetes, 132; diet for, 89, 91-92; essential, 89; exercise and, 109; eye examination for, 141; in kidneys, 30, 88; medication for, 89-93, 162; overweight and, 89
Hyperthyroidism, 139, 141, 218
Hyperventilation (overbreathing), 18
Hypothyroidism, 140, 218

Inderal (propranolol), 71, 161-64
Indomethacin, 61

Inheritance: environmental factors and, 83-84; of heart disease, 83-84
Insulin, 133-34, 136, 157
Insurance, disability, 66; *see also* Social Security
International Association for Medical Assistance to Travelers, 74
Intra-aortic balloon, 46, 53
Ischemic pericarditis, 46, 218
Isometric activity, 68-69, 219

Jogging, 64, 68, 117, 118
Johnson, Lyndon B., 80, 188
Jude, James, 44

Kidneys: arteries in, 30, 88; in heart failure, 197; infection of, 88
Kouwenhoven, William B., 44

Legs: atherosclerosis in, 30; blood clots in, 72-73, 85, 171; intra-aortic balloon in artery, 46
Leukocytes, 50, 166
Lidocaine, 45
Lipids, in blood, 28, 77, 83, 85, 213; exercise and, 108-9; hyperlipemia, 96; medication for high levels of, 100-101; purposes of, 95-96; as risk factors, 93-96; testing, 95
Lipoproteins, high-density (HDLs) and low-density (LDLs), 94-95, 107, 120, 203-4, 219
Lown, Bernard, 44
Lungs: blood circulation in, 25; blood clot in (pulmonary embolus), 42; cancer, 77, 119; collapsed (pneumothorax), 42; in heart failure, 197; pulmonary edema, 53; smoking harmful to, 77, 119-20
Lupus, drug-induced, 166

Mammary artery, 181
Medical care (attention): delay in asking for, 36-37; emergency, in heart attack, 35-37, 41-42; in foreign countries, 74; *see also* Hospital
Medication, *see* Drugs
Meralluride, 155
Mercaptomerin, 155
METS in measurement of energy, 65
Mouth-to-mouth resuscitation, 190-91, 193

INDEX

Murmurs, heart, 142

National Heart, Lung and Blood Institute, 184
National Institutes of Health, 127, 178
Neurosis, cardiac, 20
New York City Heath Department, 121
Nicotine, effects of, 77, 120
Nicotinic acid, 101
Nitroglycerin, 34, 60-61, 157-61, 220; for angina, 32, 67, 157-61; for cardiospasm, 16; exercise and, 63, 69-70, 118; propranolol with, 162; sexual activity and, 71; side effects of, 159
Norpace (Disopyramide), 167
Nuclear scanning of heart, 146-47, 220

Old age: aggression in, 115; exercise in, 113-16
Overbreathing (hyperventilation), 18
Overweight, 28, 83-84; dangers of, 101-2; in diabetes, 132, 133; exercise for reducing, 107-8; hypertension and, 89, 101; mortality in, 102; reducing diets, 103-5, *see also* Diet; as risk factor, 83, 89, 101-5; triglyceride levels in, 99-100
Oxygen: in heart attack, 46, 48; in shock, 53

Pacemakers, 220; electronic, 174-76; natural, 26, 40, 174
Pain, *see* Angina; Chest pain
Palpation, 141
Pericarditis, 61; ischemic, 46
Personality: as risk factor, 28, 83; type A, 125-30; type B, 125-28; of women, 126, 128
Phenobarbitol, 170
Phlebitis, 72-73, 85, 171, 221
Physician, choice of, 194
Pill, the, *see* Birth control pills
Plaques in atherosclerosis, 27, 202, 221
Pleurisy, 16
Pneumothorax, 42
Polythiazide, 155
Postmyocardial infarction syndrome, 61, 221
Potassium: deficiency with diuretics and digitalis, 156-57; low levels of, 91
Pregnancy: anticoagulants in, 168; avoiding, 71; echocardiography in, 146
Probenecid, 131

Procainamide (Pronestyl), 165-67, 221
Propranolol (Inderal), 71, 161-64, 221
Protamine sulphate, 169
Prothrombin, 168
Public Health Service, U.S., 79, 121, 200, 250, 255
Pulmonary artery, 25, 222
Pulmonary edema, 53
Pulmonary embolus, 42, 222
Pulmonary vein, 197, 222
Pulse, 139-40, 163, 222
Pulse deficit, 139
Pump failure, 204

Quinidine, 164-65

Radioactive isotope scanning of heart, 146-47
Randolph, Jennings, 113
Relaxation response, 92
Resuscitation: cardiopulmonary, 189-93; mouth-to-mouth, 190-91, 193
Ribs, chest pain from, 16, 17
Risk factors, 83-138, 222; after surgery, 186; for heart disease in children, 195

Salt: in diet, restricted, 78-79, 91-92, 197, 198, 204, 242-43; diuretics and, 156-57; in drinking water, 136
Saphenous vein graft, 182-83
Sedentary living: exercise program for, 116-19; and mortality from heart disease, 112; in old age, exercise for, 114-16; as risk factor, 28, 106-19
Selye, Hans, 123
Seventh-Day Adventists, 121
Sex hormones, 96
Sexual activity after heart attack, 70-72, 188
Shingles, 16
Shock, 52-53
Skin temperature, 141
Smoking, 28, 30, 77-78, 196, 200-201; atherosclerosis and, 202; giving up, 78, 121-22, 202, 244-56; heart disease and, 119-21; personality types and, 128; pipes and cigars, 121; as risk factor, 82-86, 95, 119-22; by women, 77-78, 82, 120-21
Social life, 76
Social Security, 66, 194
Sodium, 223; in diet, *see* Salt; in drinking water, 136

Spironolactone, 155
Stairs, climbing, 62-63, 68
Starch, *see* Carbohydrates
Stethoscope, 142, 223
Stress: exercise and, 109-10, 112; heart attack caused by, 124; personality type-A and, 125-30; as risk factor, 83, 122-30; work as cause, 124
Stress test, 62, 66, 145, 223
Stroke, 30, 69, 223; hypertension in, 88, 93
Sugar: in diabetes, 133-34, 136; in diet, 99-101, 136-37
Sulfinpyrazone, 131
Surgeon, choice of, 185-86
Surgery, bypass, 213, *see also* Coronary bypass; open-heart, 220; *see also* Transplants
Swimming, 63-64, 68, 117

Tachycardia, ventricular, 40
Tension: exercise and, 109-10; in old age, 115; *see also* Stress
Theophylline, 155
Thyroid gland, functioning, 139-41
Tomkins, Silvan, 249
Transcendental meditation, 92
Transplants, heart, 206-8
Travel, 72-74
Trichlormethiazide, 155
Triglycerides, 76, 79, 83, 93-95, 224; levels in blood, 94, 96, 99-100

Ultrasonic waves in echocardiography, 146
Uric acid: diuretics and, 157; as risk factor, 28, 83, 130-31

Vacations, 74-75; traveling, 73-74
Ventricles, 25, 196-97, 225
Ventricular fibrillation, 40, 43-45
Ventricular tachycardia, 40
Veterans Administration, 93
Vineberg, Arthur, 181
Vitamin E, 173-74

Walking, 64, 68, 109, 116-18; calorie expenditure in, 108
Water: drinking, 134-36; hard, 134-35
Weakness after heart attack, 49, 60
Weight: desirable, 102-3, 226; excessive, *see* Overweight
Work: after meals, 64, 68, 69; isometric activity in, 68; household, 67-69; METS in measurement of energy cost, 65; outdoors, 68, 69; physical activity and, 106-7; return to, 65-67, 187-88; stress caused by, 124
Workmen's compensation for heart attack, 193-94

X ray in heart attack, 41-42

Zoll, Paul M., 44